ESSENTIALS OF
MEDICAL STATISTICS

TO TOM

ESSENTIALS OF

Medical Statistics

BETTY R. KIRKWOOD MA MSc
Senior Lecturer in Communicable Diseases Epidemiology
(Formerly Lecturer in Medical Statistics)
London School of Hygiene and Tropical Medicine
University of London

OXFORD
Blackwell Scientific Publications
LONDON EDINBURGH BOSTON
MELBOURNE PARIS BERLIN VIENNA

Editorial Offices:
Osney Mead, Oxford OX2 0EL
25 John Street, London WC1N 2BL
23 Ainslie Place, Edinburgh EH3 6AJ
238 Main Street, Cambridge
Massachusetts 02142, USA
54 University Street, Carlton
Victoria 3053, Australia

Other Editorial Offices:
Librairie Arnette SA
2, rue Casimir-Delavigne
75006 Paris
France

Blackwell Wissenschafts-Verlag
Meinekestrasse 4
D-1000 Berlin 15
Germany

Blackwell MZV
Feldgasse 13
A-1238 Wien
Austria

First published 1988
Reprinted 1989, 1990, 1991, 1992 (twice)

Set by
Macmillan India Ltd,
Bangalore, and printed and bound
in Great Britain by Biddles Ltd,
Guildford and King's Lynn

DISTRIBUTORS
Marston Book Services Ltd
PO Box 87
Oxford OX2 0DT
(*Orders:* Tel: 0865 791155
Fax: 0865 791927
Telex: 837515)

USA
Blackwell Scientific Publications, Inc.
238 Main Street
Cambridge, MA 02142
(*Orders:* Tel: (800) 759-6102
(617) 876-7000)

Canada
Times Mirror Professional Publishing Ltd
5240 Finch Avenue East
Scarborough, Ontario M1S 5A2
(*Orders:* Tel: (800) 268-4178
(416) 298-1588)

Australia
Blackwell Scientific Publications
(Australia) Pty Ltd
54 University Street
Carlton, Victoria 3053
(*Orders:* Tel: (03) 347 0300)

British Library
Cataloguing in Publication Data

Kirkwood, Betty R.
Essentials of medical statistics.
1. Medical statistics
I. Title
610′.212 RA407

ISBN 0-632-01052-5

Contents

Preface

The aim in writing this book has been to put the multitude of statistical methods applicable to medical research into their practical context, and in doing this I hope I have combined simplicity with depth. I have adopted a somewhat different ordering of topics than found in most books, based on a logical progression of practical concepts, rather than a formal mathematical development. Statistical ideas are introduced as and when needed, and all methods are described in the context of relevant examples drawn from real situations. There is extensive cross-referencing to link and contrast the alternative approaches which may apply in similar situations. In this way the reader is led more quickly to the analysis of practical problems and should find it easier to learn which procedures are applicable when.

This book is suitable for self-instruction, as a companion to lecture courses on medical statistics, and as a reference text. It covers all topics which a medical research worker or student is likely to encounter. Some advanced (or uncommon) methods are described only briefly, and the reader referred to more specialist books. It is hoped, however, that it will be a rare event to look for a topic in the index, and not to find even a mention. All formulae are clearly highlighted for easy reference, and there is a useful summary of methods on the inside front and back covers.

The book is a concise and straightforward introduction to the basic methods and ideas of medical statistics. It does not, however, stop here. It is intended also to be a reasonably comprehensive guide to the subject. For anyone seriously involved in statistical applications, it is not sufficient just to be able to carry out, for example, a *t* test. It is also important to appreciate the limitations of the simple methods, and to know when and how they should be extended. For this reason, chapters have been included on, for example, analysis of variance and multiple regression. When dealing with these more advanced methods the treatment concentrates on the principles involved and the interpretation of results, since with the wide availability of computing facilities it is no longer necessary to acquire familiarity with the details of the calculations. The more advanced sections may be omitted at a first reading, as indicated at the relevant points in the text. It is recommended, however, that the introductions of all chapters are read, as these put the different methods into context.

The reader will also find such topics as trend tests for contingency tables, methods of standardization, use of transformations, survival analysis and case–control studies. The last quarter of the book is devoted to issues involved in the design and conduct of investigations. These sections are not divorced in any way from the sections on methods of analysis and reflect the importance of an awareness of statistics throughout the execution of a study. There is a detailed summary of how to decide on an appropriate sample size, and an introduction to the use of computers, with much of the common jargon explained.

This book has been compiled from several years' experience both of teaching statistics to a variety of medical personnel and of collaborative research. I hope that the approach I have adopted will appeal to anyone working in or associated with the field of medical research, and will please medical workers and statisticians alike. In particular, I hope the result will answer the expressed need of many that the problem in carrying out statistical work is not so much learning the mechanics of a particular test, but rather knowing which method to apply when.

I would like to express my gratitude to the many colleagues, students, and friends who have assisted me in this task. In particular, I would like to thank David Ross and Cesar Victora for willingly reading early drafts and commenting in great detail, Richard Hayes for many discussions on teaching over the years, Laura Rodrigues for sharing her insight into epidemiological methodology with me, Peter Smith for comments and general support, Helen Edwards for patient and skilled help with the typing, and Jacqui Wright for assistance in compiling the appendix tables. I would also like to thank my husband Tom Kirkwood not only for comments on many drafts, endless discussions and practical help, but also for providing unfailing support and encouragement throughout. It is to him this book is dedicated. Finally, I would like to mention Daisy and Sam Kirkwood, whose birth, although delaying the finalization of an almost complete manuscript, provided me with an opportunity to take a fresh look at what I had written and make a number of major improvements.

CHAPTER 1

Basics

What is statistics?

Statistics is the science of collecting, summarizing, presenting, and interpreting data, and of using them to test hypotheses. During the last few decades it has assumed an increasingly central role in medical investigations. The reasons for this are many, three of the principal ones being as follows. Firstly, statistics provides a way of organizing information on a wider and more formal basis than relying on the exchange of anecdotes and personal experience. Secondly, more and more things are now measured quantitatively in medicine. Thirdly, there is a great deal of intrinsic variation in most biological processes. For example, not only does blood pressure differ from person to person, but in the same person it also varies from day to day and from hour to hour. It is the interpretation of data in the presence of such variability that lies at the heart of statistics. Thus, in investigating morbidity associated with a particular stressful occupation, statistical methods would be needed to assess whether an observed average blood pressure above that of the general population could simply be due to chance variations or whether it represents a real indication of an occupational health risk.

Variability can also arise through the random operation of chance within a population. Individuals do not all react in the same way to a given stimulus. Thus, although smoking and drinking are in general bad for the health, one not infrequently hears of a heavy smoker and drinker living to healthy old age, whereas a non-smoking teetotaller may die young. As another example, consider the evaluation of a new vaccine. Individuals vary both in their responsiveness to vaccines and in their susceptibility and exposure to disease. Not only will some people who are unvaccinated escape infection, but also a number of those who are vaccinated may contract the disease. What can be concluded if the percentage of people free from the disease is greater among the vaccinated group than among the unvaccinated? Is the vaccine really effective? Could the results just be due to chance? Or, was there some bias in the way people were selected for vaccination, for example were they of different ages or social class, such that their risk of contracting the disease was in any case lower? The methods of statistical analysis are used to discriminate between the first two of these possibilities, while the choice of an appropriate design should exclude the third. This example illustrates that the usefulness of statistics is not confined to the analysis of results. It also has a role to play in the design and conduct of a study.

Populations and samples

Associated with the basic issue of variability is the important point that, except when a full census is taken, the data are for a **sample** from a much larger group called the **population**. The sample is of interest not in its own right, but for what it tells the investigator about the population. Because of chance, different samples give different results and this must be taken into account when using a sample to make inferences about the population. This phenomenon, called **sampling variation**, lies at the heart of statistics. It is described in detail in Chapter 3.

The word 'population' is used in statistics in a wider sense than usual. It is not limited to a population of people but can refer to any collection of objects. For example, the data may relate to a sample of 20 hospitals from the population of all hospitals in the country. In such a case it is easy to imagine that the entire population can be listed and the sample selected directly from it. In many instances, however, the population and its boundaries are less precisely specified, and care must be taken to ensure that the sample truly represents the population about which information is required. This population is sometimes referred to as the **target population**. For example, consider a vaccine trial carried out using student volunteers. If it is reasonable to assume that in their response to the vaccine and exposure to disease students are typical of the community at large, the results will have general applicability. If, on the other hand, students differ in any respect which may materially affect their response to the vaccine or exposure to disease, the conclusions from the trial are restricted to the population of students and do not have general applicability. In this instance, the target population includes not only all persons living at present but also those that may be alive at some time in the future. It is obvious that the complete enumeration of such a population is not possible.

Defining the data

The raw data of an investigation consist of **observations** made on individuals. In many situations the individuals are people, but they need not be. For instance, they might be red blood cells, urine specimens, rats, or hospitals. The number of individuals is called the **sample size**. Any aspect of an individual that is measured, like blood pressure, or recorded, like age or sex, is called a **variable**. There may be only one variable in a study or there may be many.

It is helpful to divide variables into different types as different statistical methods are applicable to each. The main division is into **qualitative** (or **categorical**) and **quantitative** (or **numerical**) variables. A qualitative variable is non-numerical, for instance place of birth, ethnic group, or type of drug. A particularly common sort is a **binary** variable, where the response is one of two alternatives. For example, sex is male or female, or a patient survives or dies. A quantitative variable is numerical and either **discrete** or **continuous**. The values of a discrete variable are usually whole numbers, such as the number of cases of pertussis in a week. A continuous variable, as the name implies, is a measurement on a continuous scale. Examples are height, weight, blood pressure, and age.

Data analysis and presentation of results

The methods of summarizing and analysing data in order to interpret the results of a study form the basis of this book. Three general points deserve emphasis here. The first is that the application of complex methods for their own sake should be avoided. It is important to start by using basic summary and graphical techniques to explore the data. The analysis should then progress from the simple to the complex. The method chosen should be the simplest consistent with the requirements of the data.

The second and related point is that statistical reasoning should be applied hand in hand with common sense. It is important not to lose sight of the numbers themselves, the factors influencing them, and what they stand for while manipulating them in the midst of an analysis. Bradford Hill (1977), Colton (1974), and Oldham (1968) all have useful chapters illustrating the common fallacies and difficulties that arise in the interpretation of data.

The third point is that **graphical techniques** are strongly recommended, both during the exploratory phase of an analysis and for the presentation of results, since relationships, trends, and contrasts are often more readily appreciated from a diagram than from a table. Diagrams (and tables) should always be clearly labelled and self-explanatory; it should not be necessary to refer to the text to understand them. At the same time they should not be cluttered with too much detail, and they must not be misleading. Breaks and discontinuities in the scale(s) should be clearly marked, and avoided whenever possible. Figure 1.1(a) shows a common form of misrepresentation due to an inappropriate use of scale. The decline in infant mortality rate (IMR) has been made to look dramatic by expanding the vertical scale, while in reality the decrease over the 10 years displayed is only slight (from 22.7 to 22.1

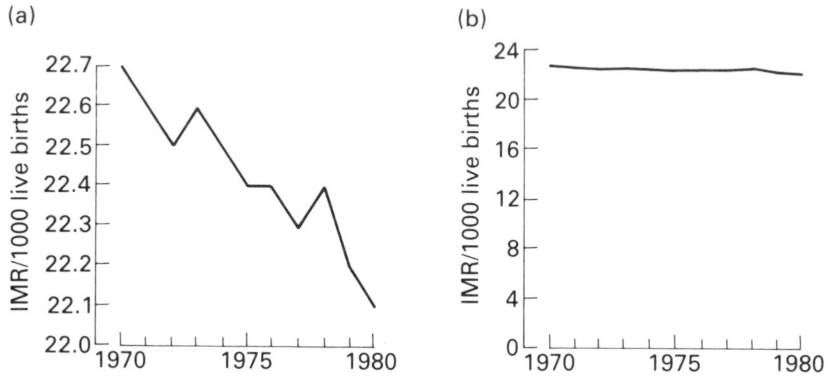

Figure 1.1 Decline in infant mortality rate (IMR) between 1970 and 1980. (a) Inappropriate choice of scale has misleadingly exaggerated the decline. (b) Correct use of scale.

deaths/1000 livebirths/year). A more realistic representation is shown in Figure 1.1(b), with the vertical scale starting at zero.

Choice of a calculator

A calculator is essential for even the simplest of statistical applications. There are a wide variety of different machines available covering a wide price range. The following facilities are recommended as a minimum.

1 Scientific functions such as square root, logarithm, and factorial.
2 At least one memory.
3 Automatic calculation of mean and standard deviation.
4 Automatic calculation of correlation and linear regression.
5 A programming facility, with the capacity to store at least 100 programming steps, which remain when the calculator is turned off. This capacity should be sufficient to allow two programs to be resident in the calculator to cover the two most commonly used statistical tests, a *t* test to compare two means (*see* Chapter 7) and a chi-squared test to compare two proportions (*see* Chapter 13).

It is possible to find a relatively inexpensive calculator (about £20) satisfying all these conditions. The main benefits to be gained from more expensive machines are an increase in the number of programming steps and the ability to store additional programs on external media, such as a magnetic strip or audio-cassette.

CHAPTER 2

Frequencies, Frequency Distributions, and Histograms

Introduction

The first step of an analysis is to summarize the data, since data which have not been organized in any way are not very easy to understand. It often helps to illustrate them with a diagram, which should always be clearly labelled and self-explanatory.

Frequencies (qualitative data)

Summarizing qualitative data is very straightforward, the main task being to count the number of observations in each category. These counts are called **frequencies**. They are often also presented as **relative frequencies**, that is as percentages of the total number of individuals. For example, Table 2.1 summarizes the method of delivery recorded for 600 births in a hospital. The variable of interest is the method of delivery, a qualitative variable with three categories, normal delivery, forceps delivery, and caesarean section.

Table 2.1 Method of delivery of 600 babies born in a hospital.

Method of delivery	No. of births	Percentage
Normal	478	79.7
Forceps	65	10.8
Caesarean section	57	9.5
Total	600	100.0

Frequencies and relative frequencies are commonly illustrated by a **bar diagram** (*see* Figure 2.1) or by a **pie chart** (*see* Figure 2.2). In a bar diagram the lengths of the bars are drawn proportional to the frequencies, and in a pie chart the circle is divided so that the areas of the sectors are proportional to the frequencies.

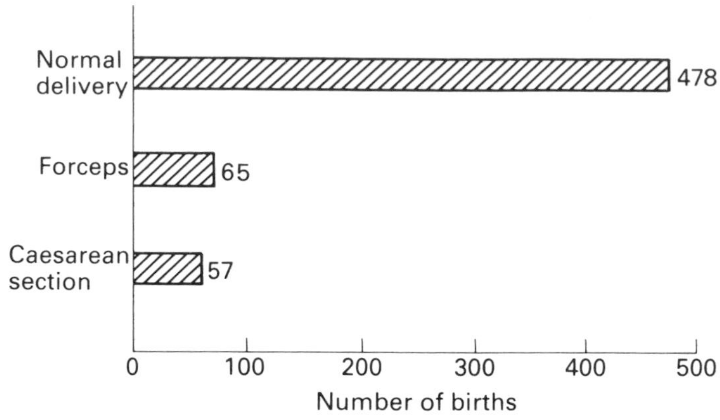

Figure 2.1 Bar diagram showing method of delivery of 600 babies born in a hospital.

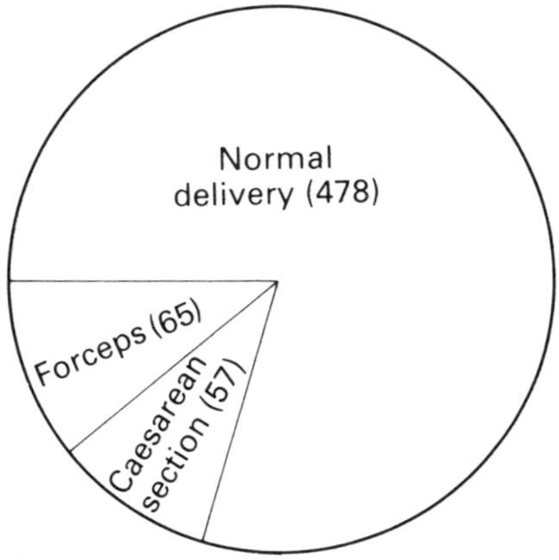

Figure 2.2 Pie chart showing method of delivery of 600 babies born in a hospital.

Frequency distributions (quantitative data)

If there are more than about 20 observations, a useful first step in summarizing quantitative data is to form a **frequency distribution**. This is a table showing the number of observations at different values or within certain ranges. For a discrete variable the frequencies may be tabulated either for each value of the variable or for groups of values. With continuous variables, groups have to be formed. An example is given in Table 2.2, where haemoglobin has been measured to the nearest 0.1 g/100 ml and the group 11–, for example, contains all measurements between 11.0 and 11.9 g/100 ml inclusive.

Table 2.2 Haemoglobin levels in g/100 ml for 70 women.

(a) Raw data (the lowest and highest values are underlined).

10.2	13.7	10.4	14.9	11.5	12.0	11.0
13.3	12.9	12.1	9.4	13.2	10.8	11.7
10.6	10.5	13.7	11.8	14.1	10.3	13.6
12.1	12.9	11.4	12.7	10.6	11.4	11.9
9.3	13.5	14.6	11.2	11.7	10.9	10.4
12.0	12.9	11.1	8.8	10.2	11.6	12.5
13.4	12.1	10.9	11.3	14.7	10.8	13.3
11.9	11.4	12.5	13.0	11.6	13.1	9.7
11.2	15.1	10.7	12.9	13.4	12.3	11.0
14.6	11.1	13.5	10.9	13.1	11.8	12.2

(b) Frequency distribution.

Haemoglobin (g/100 ml)	Tally	No. of women	Percentage
8–	1	1	1.4
9–	111	3	4.3
10–	~~1111~~ ~~1111~~ 1111	14	20.0
11–	~~1111~~ ~~1111~~ ~~1111~~ 1111	19	27.1
12–	~~1111~~ ~~1111~~ 1111	14	20.0
13–	~~1111~~ ~~1111~~ 1111	13	18.6
14–	~~1111~~	5	7.1
15–15.9	1	1	1.4
Total		70	100.0

When forming a frequency distribution, the first things to do are to count the number of observations and to identify the lowest and highest values. Then decide whether the data should be grouped, and, if so, what grouping interval should be used. As a rough guide one should aim for 5–20 groups, depending on the number of observations. If the interval chosen for grouping the data is too wide, too much detail will be lost, while if it is too narrow the table will be unwieldy. The starting points of the groups should be round numbers and, whenever possible, all the intervals should be of the same width. There should be no gaps between groups. The table should be labelled so that it is clear what happens to observations that fall on the boundaries.

For example, in Table 2.2 there are 70 haemoglobin measurements. The lowest value is 8.8 and the highest 15.1 g/100 ml. Intervals of width 1 g/100 ml were chosen, leading to eight groups in the frequency distribution. Labelling the groups 8–, 9–, . . . is clear. An acceptable alternative would have been 8.0–8.9, 9.0–9.9 and so on. Note that labelling them 8–9, 9–10 and so on would have been confusing, since it would not then be clear to which group a measurement of 9.0 g/100 ml, for example, belonged.

Once the format of the table is decided, the numbers of observations in each group are counted. Mistakes are most easily avoided by going through the data in order. For each value, a mark is put against the appropriate group. To facilitate the counting, these marks are arranged in groups of five by putting each fifth mark horizontally through the previous four (~~||||~~); these are called **five-bar gates**. The process is called **tallying** and is illustrated in Table 2.2(b).

Histograms

Frequency distributions are usually illustrated by histograms, as shown in Figure 2.3 for the haemoglobin data. Either the frequencies or the percentages may be used; the shape of the histogram will be the same.

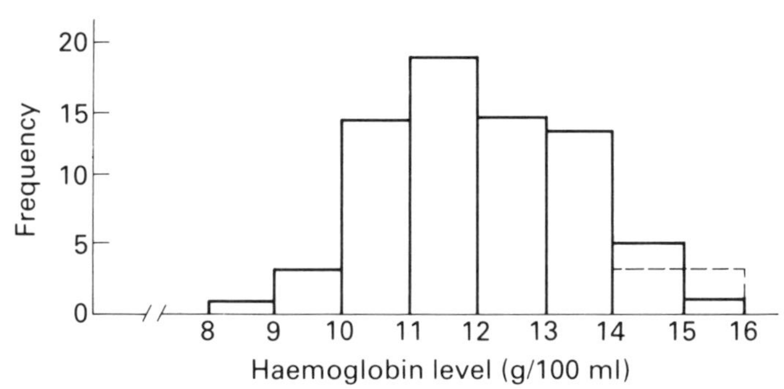

Figure 2.3 Histogram of haemoglobin levels of 70 women.

The construction of a histogram is straightforward when the grouping intervals of the frequency distribution are all equal, as is the case in Figure 2.3. If the intervals are of different widths, it is important to take this into account when drawing the histogram, otherwise a distorted picture will be obtained. For example, suppose the two highest haemoglobin groups had been combined in compiling Table 2.2(b). The frequency for this combined group (14.0–15.9 g/100 ml) would be 6, but clearly it would be misleading to draw a rectangle of height 6 from 14 to 16 g/100 ml. Since this interval would be *twice* the width of all the others, the correct height of the line would be 3, *half* the total frequency for this group. This is illustrated by the dotted line in Figure 2.3. The general rule for drawing a histogram when the intervals are not all the same width is to make the heights of the rectangles proportional to the frequencies divided by the widths, that is to make the *areas* of the histogram bars proportional to the frequencies.

Frequency polygon

An alternative but less common way of illustrating a frequency distribution is a frequency polygon, as shown in Figure 2.4. This is particularly useful when comparing two or more frequency distributions by drawing them on the same diagram. The polygon is drawn by imagining (or lightly pencilling) the histogram and joining the mid-points of the tops of its rectangles. The end-points of the resulting line are then joined to the horizontal axis at the mid-points of the groups immediately below and above the lowest and highest non-zero frequencies respectively. For the haemoglobin data, these are the groups 7.0–7.9 and 16.0–16.9 g/100 ml. The frequency polygon in Figure 2.4 is therefore joined to the axis at 7.5 and 16.5 g/100 ml.

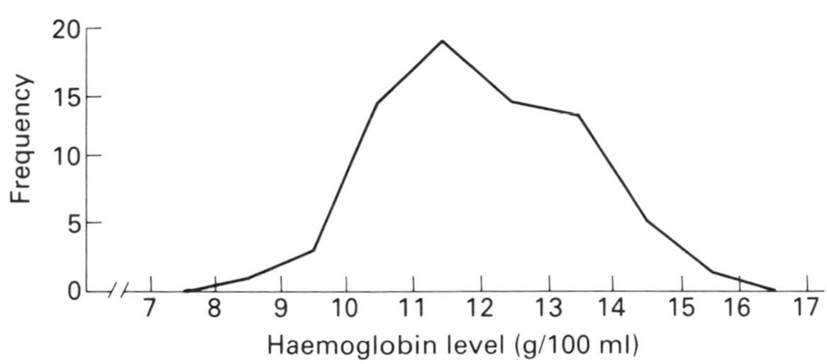

Figure 2.4 Frequency polygon of haemoglobin levels of 70 women.

Frequency distribution of the population

Figures 2.3 and 2.4 illustrate the frequency distribution of the haemoglobin levels of a sample of 70 women. We use these data to give us information about the distribution of haemoglobin levels among women in general. For example, it seems uncommon for a woman to have a level below 9.0 g/100 ml or above 15.0 g/100 ml. Our confidence in drawing general conclusions from the data depends on how many individuals were measured. The larger the sample measured, the finer the grouping interval that can be chosen, so that the histogram (or frequency polygon) becomes smoother and more closely resembles the distribution of the total population. In the limit, if it were possible to ascertain the haemoglobin levels of the whole population of women, the resulting diagram would be a smooth curve.

Shapes of frequency distributions

Figure 2.5 shows three of the most common shapes of frequency distributions. They all have high frequencies in the centre of the distribution and low frequencies at the two extremes, which are called the **upper** and **lower tails** of the distribution. The distribution in Figure 2.5(a) is also **symmetrical** about the centre; this shape of curve is often described as 'bell-shaped'. The two other distributions are asymmetrical or **skewed**. The upper tail of the distribution in Figure 2.5(b) is longer than the lower tail; this is called positively skewed or skewed to the right. The distribution in Figure 2.5(c) is negatively skewed or skewed to the left.

All three distributions in Figure 2.5 are **unimodal**, that is they have just one peak. Figure 2.6(a) shows a **bimodal** frequency distribution, that is a

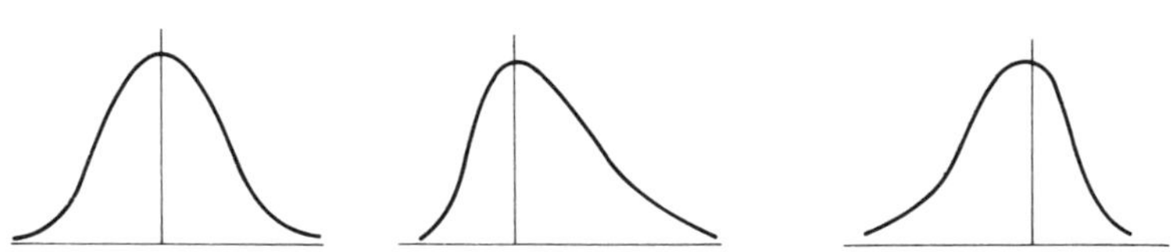

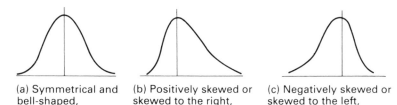

(a) Symmetrical and bell-shaped, e.g. height

(b) Positively skewed or skewed to the right, e.g. triceps skinfold measurement

(c) Negatively skewed or skewed to the left, e.g. period of gestation

Figure 2.5 Three common shapes of frequency distributions with an example of each.

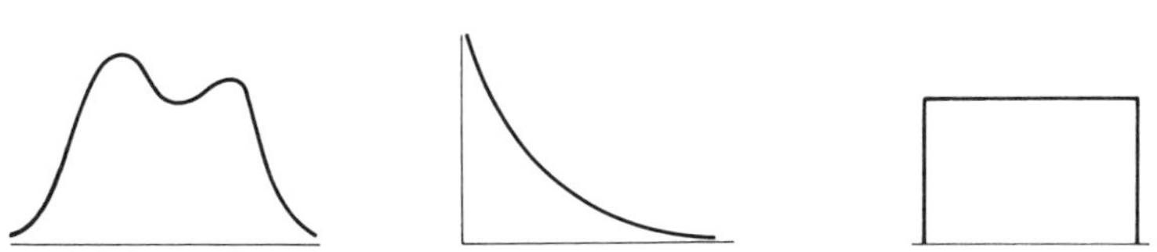

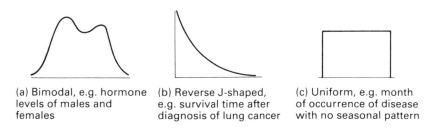

(a) Bimodal, e.g. hormone levels of males and females

(b) Reverse J-shaped, e.g. survival time after diagnosis of lung cancer

(c) Uniform, e.g. month of occurrence of disease with no seasonal pattern

Figure 2.6 Three less common shapes of frequency distributions with an example of each.

distribution with two peaks. This is occasionally seen and usually indicates that the data are a mixture of two separate distributions. Also shown in Figure 2.6 are two other distributions that are sometimes found; the **reverse J-shaped** and the **uniform** distributions.

CHAPTER 3

Means, Standard Deviations, and Standard Errors

Introduction

A frequency distribution gives a general picture of the values of a variable. It is often convenient, however, to summarize a quantitative variable still further by giving just two measurements, one indicating the average value and the other the spread of the values.

Mean, median, and mode

The average value is usually represented by the **arithmetic mean**, customarily just called the mean. This is simply the sum of the values divided by the number of values.

$$\text{Mean, } \bar{x} = \frac{\Sigma x}{n}$$

where x denotes the values of the variable, Σ (the Greek capital letter sigma) means 'the sum of' and n is the number of observations. The mean is denoted by $\bar{x}$ (spoken 'x bar').

Other measures of the average value are the **median** and the **mode**. The median is the value that divides the distribution in half. If the observations are arranged in increasing order, the median is the middle observation.

$$\text{Median} = \frac{(n+1)}{2} \text{ th value of ordered observations}$$

If there is an even number of observations, there is no middle one and the average of the two 'middle' ones is taken. The **mode** is the value which occurs most often.

Example 3.1
The following are the plasma volumes of eight healthy adult males:

2.75, 2.86, 3.37, 2.76, 2.62, 3.49, 3.05, 3.12 litres

(a) $n=8$

$\Sigma x = 2.75+2.86+3.37+2.76+2.62+3.49+3.05+3.12 = 24.02$ l

Mean, $\bar{x} = \Sigma x/n = 24.02/8 = 3.00$ l

(b) Rearranging the measurements in increasing order gives:

2.62, 2.75, 2.76, 2.86, 3.05, 3.12, 3.37, 3.49 l

Median $=(n+1)/2 = 9/2 = 4\frac{1}{2}$ th value

$=$ average of 4th and 5th values

$=(2.86+3.05)/2 = 2.96$ l

(c) There is no estimate of the mode, since all the values are different.

The mean is usually the preferred measure since it takes into account each individual observation and is most amenable to mathematical and statistical techniques. The median is a useful descriptive measure if there are one or two extremely high or low values, which would make the mean unrepresentative of the majority of the data. The mode is seldom used. If the sample is small, either it may not be possible to estimate the mode (as in Example 3.1c), or the estimate obtained may be misleading. The mean, median and mode are, *on average*, equal, however, when the distribution is symmetrical and unimodal. When the distribution is positively skewed, a **geometric mean** is more appropriate than the arithmetic mean. This is discussed in Chapter 19.

Measures of variation

The simplest measure of variation is the **range**, which is the difference between the largest and smallest values. Its disadvantage is that it is based on only two of the observations and gives no idea of how the other observations are arranged between these two. Also, it tends to be larger, the larger the size of the sample.

Since the variation is small if the observations are bunched closely about their mean, and large if they are scattered over considerable distances, variation is measured instead in terms of the deviations of the observations from the mean. The **variance** is the average of the *squares* of these differences. When calculating the variance of a sample, the sum of squared deviations is divided by $(n-1)$ rather than n, however, because this gives a better estimate of the variance of the total population.

$$\text{Variance, } s^2 = \frac{\Sigma(x-\bar{x})^2}{(n-1)}$$

Degrees of freedom

The denominator $(n-1)$ is called the number of **degrees of freedom** of the variance. This number is $(n-1)$ rather than n, since only $(n-1)$ of the deviations $(x-\bar{x})$ are independent from each other. The last one can always be calculated from the others because all n of them must add up to zero.

Standard deviation

The variance has convenient mathematical properties and is the appropriate measure when doing statistical theory. A disadvantage, however, is that it is in the *square* of the units used for the observations. For example, if the observations are weights in grams, the variance is in grams squared. For many purposes it is more convenient to express the variation in the original units by taking the *square root* of the variance. This is called the **standard deviation** (s.d.).

$$\text{s.d., } s=\sqrt{\left[\frac{\Sigma(x-\bar{x})^2}{(n-1)}\right]}$$

or equivalently

$$s=\sqrt{\left[\frac{\Sigma x^2-(\Sigma x)^2/n}{(n-1)}\right]}$$

The latter is a more convenient form for calculation, since the mean does not have to be calculated first and then subtracted from each of the observations. The equivalence of the two formulae is demonstrated in Example 3.2. (Note: Many calculators have built-in functions for the mean and standard deviation. The keys are commonly labelled $\bar{x}$ and σ_{n-1}, respectively, where σ is the lower case Greek letter sigma.)

Example 3.2

Table 3.1 shows the steps for the calculation of the standard deviation of the eight plasma volume measurements of Example 3.1. Note that

$$\Sigma x^2-(\Sigma x)^2/n=72.7980-(24.02)^2/8=0.6780$$

gives the same answer as $\Sigma(x-\bar{x})^2$:

$$s=\sqrt{(0.6780/7)}=0.311$$

Table 3.1 Calculation of the standard deviation of the plasma volumes (l) of eight healthy adult males (same data as in Example 3.1). Mean, $\bar{x} = 3.00$ l.

	Plasma volume (l) x	Deviation from the mean $x - \bar{x}$	Squared deviation $(x - \bar{x})^2$	Squared observation x^2
	2.75	−0.25	0.0625	7.5625
	2.86	−0.14	0.0196	8.1796
	3.37	0.37	0.1369	11.3569
	2.76	−0.24	0.0576	7.6176
	2.62	−0.38	0.1444	6.8644
	3.49	0.49	0.2401	12.1801
	3.05	0.05	0.0025	9.3025
	3.12	0.12	0.0144	9.7344
Totals	24.02	0.00	0.6780	72.7980

Interpretation

Usually about 70% of the observations lie within one standard deviation of their mean, and about 95% lie within two standard deviations. These figures are based on a theoretical frequency distribution, called the normal distribution, which is described in Chapter 4.

Coefficient of variation

$$\text{c.v.} = \frac{s}{\bar{x}} \times 100\%$$

The coefficient of variation expresses the standard deviation as a percentage of the sample mean. This is useful when interest is in the size of the variation relative to the size of the observation, and it has the advantage that the coefficient of variation is independent of the units of observation. For example, the value of the standard deviation of a set of weights will be different depending on whether they are measured in kilograms or pounds. The coefficient of variation, however, will be the same in the two units.

Calculating the mean and standard deviation from a frequency distribution

Table 3.2 shows the distribution of the number of previous pregnancies of a group of women attending an antenatal clinic. Eighteen of the 100 women had no previous pregnancies, 27 had one, 31 had two, 19 had three, and 5 had four previous pregnancies. As, for example, adding 2 thirty-one times is equivalent to adding the product (2×31), the total number of previous pregnancies is calculated by:

$$\begin{aligned}\Sigma x &= (0 \times 18) + (1 \times 27) + (2 \times 31) + (3 \times 19) + (4 \times 5)\\ &= 0 + 27 + 62 + 57 + 20 = 166\end{aligned}$$

The average number of previous pregnancies is, therefore:

$$\bar{x} = 166/100 = 1.66$$

In the same way:

$$\begin{aligned}\Sigma x^2 &= (0^2 \times 18) + (1^2 \times 27) + (2^2 \times 31) + (3^2 \times 19) + (4^2 \times 5)\\ &= 0 + 27 + 124 + 171 + 80 = 402\end{aligned}$$

The standard deviation is, therefore:

$$s = \sqrt{\frac{(402 - 166^2/100)}{99}} = \sqrt{\frac{126.44}{99}} = 1.13$$

Table 3.2 Distribution of the number of previous pregnancies of a group of women aged 30–34 attending an antenatal clinic.

	No. of previous pregnancies					
	0	1	2	3	4	Total
No. of women	18	27	31	19	5	100

If a variable has been grouped when constructing a frequency distribution, its mean and standard deviation should be calculated using the original values, not the frequency distribution. There are occasions, however, when only the frequency distribution is available. In such a case, approximate values for the mean and standard deviation can be calculated by using the values of the mid-points of the groups and proceeding as above.

Change of units

Adding or subtracting a constant from the observations alters the mean by the same amount but leaves the standard deviation unaffected. Multiplying or dividing by a constant changes both the mean and the standard deviation in the same way.

For example, suppose a set of temperatures is converted from Fahrenheit to centigrade. This is done by subtracting 32, multiplying by 5, and dividing by 9. The new mean may be calculated from the old one in exactly the same way, that is by subtracting 32, multiplying by 5, and dividing by 9. The new standard deviation, however, is simply the old one multiplied by 5 and divided by 9, since the subtraction does not affect it.

Sampling variation and standard error

As discussed in Chapter 1, the sample is of interest not in its own right, but for what it tells the investigator about the population which it represents. The sample mean, $\bar{x}$, and standard deviation, s, are used to estimate the mean and standard deviation of the population, denoted by the Greek letters μ (mu) and σ (sigma) respectively. The sample mean is unlikely to be exactly equal to the population mean. A different sample would give a different estimate, the difference being due to sampling variation. Imagine collecting many independent samples of the same size and calculating the sample mean of each of them. A frequency distribution of these means could then be formed. The mean of this distribution would be the population mean, and it can be shown that its standard deviation would equal $\sigma/\sqrt{n}$. This is called the **standard error of the sample mean**, and it measures how precisely the population mean is estimated by the sample mean. The size of the standard error depends both on how much variation there is in the population and on the size of the sample. The larger the sample, the smaller is the standard error.

We seldom know the population standard deviation, σ, however, and so we use the sample standard deviation, s, to estimate the standard error.

$$\text{s.e.} = \frac{s}{\sqrt{n}}$$

Example 3.3

The mean of the eight plasma volumes shown in Table 3.1 is 3.00 l (Example 3.1) and the standard deviation is 0.31 l (Example 3.2). The standard error of the mean is therefore estimated as:

$$s/\sqrt{n}=0.31/\sqrt{8}=0.111$$

Example 3.4

Figure 3.1 shows the results of a game played with a class of 30 students to illustrate the concepts of sampling variation, the sampling distribution, and standard error. Blood pressure measurements for 250 airline pilots were used. The distribution of these measurements is shown in Figure 3.1(a). The population mean, μ, was 78.2 mmHg, and the population standard deviation, σ, was 9.4 mmHg. Each value was written on a small disc and the 250 discs put into a bag. Each student was asked to shake the bag, select 10 discs, write down the 10 diastolic blood pressures, work out their mean, $\bar{x}$, and return the discs to the bag. In this way 30 different samples were obtained, with 30 different sample means, each estimating the same population mean. The mean of these sample means was 78.23 mmHg, close to the population mean. Their distribution is shown in Figure 3.1(b). The standard deviation of the sample means was 3.01 mmHg, which agreed well with the theoretical value, $\sigma/\sqrt{n}=9.4/\sqrt{10}=2.97$ mmHg, for the standard error of the mean of a sample of size 10.

The exercise was repeated taking samples of size 20. The results are shown in Figure 3.1(c). The reduced variation in the sample means resulting from increasing the sample size from 10 to 20 can be clearly seen. The mean of the sample means was 78.14 mmHg, again close to the population mean. The standard deviation was 2.07 mmHg, again in good agreement with the theoretical value, $9.4/\sqrt{20}=2.10$ mmHg.

Interpretation

The interpretation of the standard error of a sample mean is similar to that of the standard deviation. Approximately 95% of the sample means obtained by repeated sampling would lie within two standard errors above or below the population mean. This fact can be used to construct a range of likely values for the (unknown) population mean, based on the observed sample mean and its standard error. Such a range is called a **confidence interval**. Its method of construction is not described until Chapter 5 since it depends on using the normal distribution, described in Chapter 4.

Finite population correction

If a sample is from a population of finite size, for example the houses in a village, the sampling variation is considerably smaller than $\sigma/\sqrt{n}$ when a

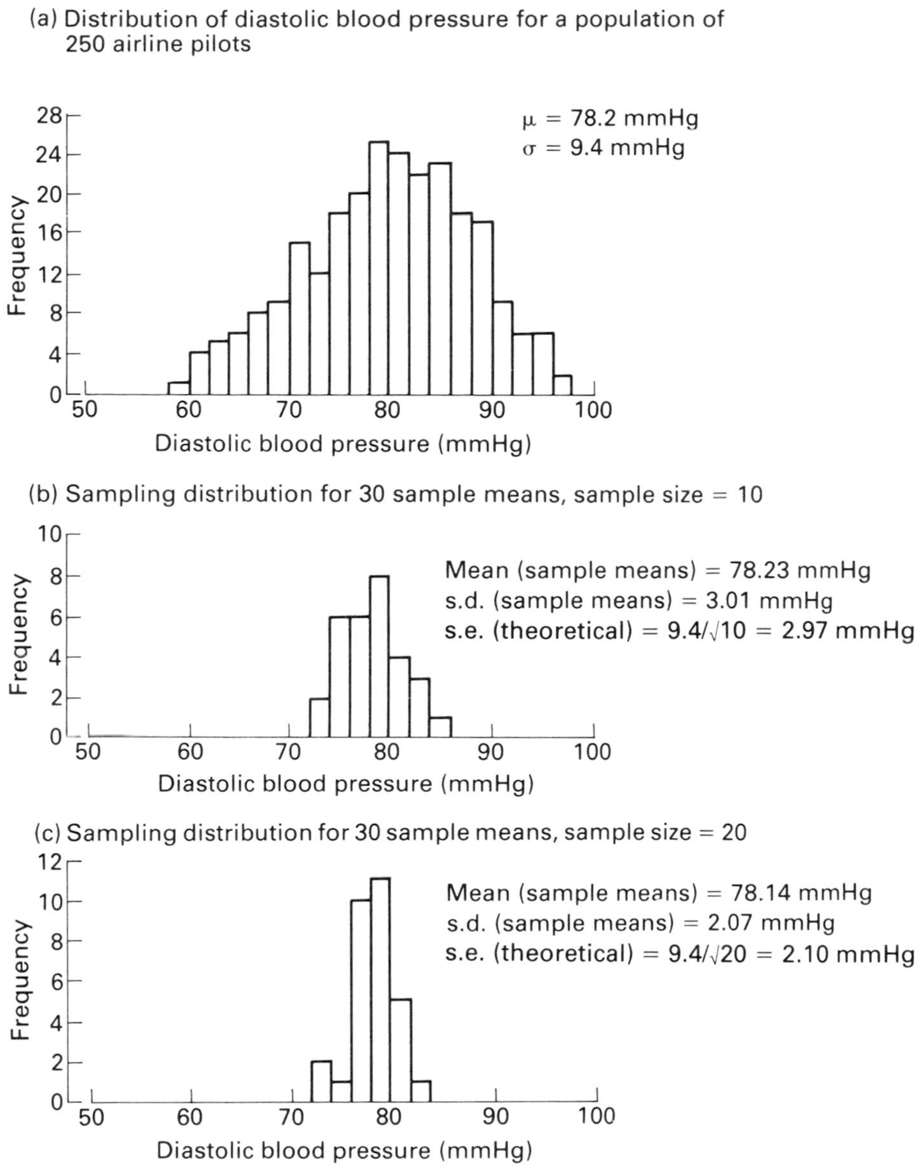

Figure 3.1 Results of a game played to illustrate the concepts of sampling variation, the sampling distribution, and the standard error.

large proportion of the population is sampled. It would be zero if the whole population were sampled, not because there is no variation among individuals in the population, but because the sample mean *is* then the population mean. A second sample of the same size (i.e. the whole population) would automatically give the same result. A **finite population correction** (f.p.c.) is therefore applied when working out the standard error. The formula becomes:

$$\text{s.e. with f.p.c.} = \frac{\sigma}{\sqrt{n}}\sqrt{\left(1-\frac{n}{N}\right)}$$

where N is the population size and n/N is the **sampling fraction**.

Ignoring the finite population correction results in an overestimation of the standard error. For example, if 75% of the population were sampled, the finite population correction would equal $\sqrt{(1-0.75)}=0.5$. If this were omitted, the standard error estimated would be twice the correct value. The correction has little effect and can be ignored when the sampling fraction is smaller than about 10%.

CHAPTER 4

The Normal Distribution

Introduction

Frequency distributions and their various shapes were discussed in Chapter 2. In practice it is found that a reasonable description of many variables is provided by the **normal distribution**, sometimes called the Gaussian distribution after its discoverer, Gauss. The curve of the normal distribution is symmetrical about the mean and bell-shaped; the bell is tall and narrow for small standard deviations and short and wide for large ones. Figure 4.1 illustrates the normal curve describing the distribution of heights of adult men in the United Kingdom. Other examples of variables that are approximately normally distributed are blood pressure, body temperature, and haemoglobin level. Examples of variables that are not normally distributed are triceps skinfold thickness and income, both of which are positively skewed. Sometimes transforming a variable, for example by taking logarithms, will make its distribution more normal. This is described in Chapter 19, and how to assess whether a variable is normally distributed is discussed in Chapter 18.

The normal distribution is important not only because it is a good empirical description of many variables, but because it occupies a central role in the techniques of statistical analysis. For example, it is the justification for the calculation of the confidence interval which was mentioned in Chapter 3

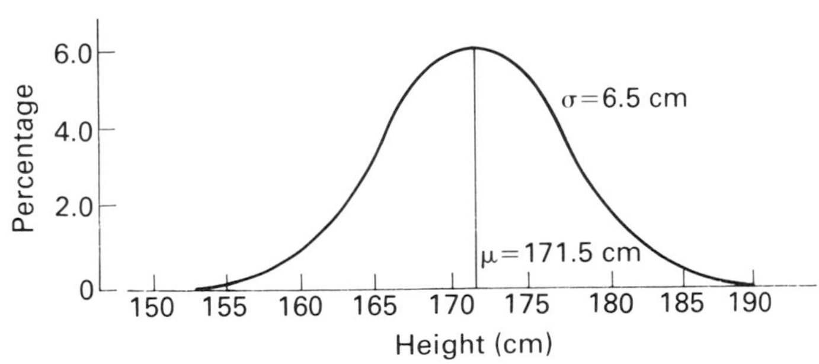

Figure 4.1 Diagram showing the approximate normal curve describing the distribution of heights of adult men.

and which is described in Chapter 5. It also forms the basis of the methodology of significance testing of means which is introduced in Chapter 6. For these reasons it is important to describe the use of the normal distribution in some detail before proceeding further, although the precise mathematical equation which defines it need not be a concern as tables are available.

The standard normal distribution

If a variable is normally distributed then a change of units does not affect this. Thus, for example, whether height is measured in centimetres or inches it is normally distributed. Changing the mean simply moves the curve up or down the axis, while changing the standard deviation alters the height and width of the curve.

In particular, by a suitable change of units any normally distributed variable can be related to the **standard normal distribution** whose mean is zero and whose standard deviation is 1. This is done by subtracting the mean from each observation and dividing by the standard deviation. The relationship is:

$$\text{SND, } z = \frac{x - \mu}{\sigma}$$

where x is the original variable with mean μ and standard deviation σ and z is

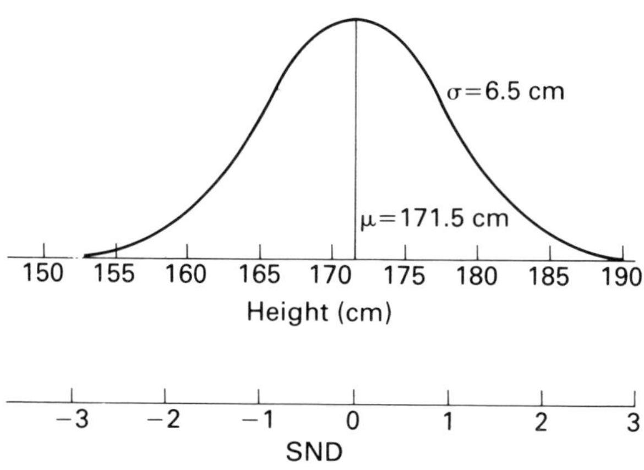

Figure 4.2 Relationship between normal distribution in original units of measurement and in standard normal deviates.

SND = (height − 171.5)/6.5
Height = 171.5 + (6.5 × SND)

the corresponding **standard normal deviate** (SND). This is illustrated for the distribution of adult male heights in Figure 4.2.

The possibility of converting any normally distributed variable into an SND means that tables are only needed for the standard normal distribution and not for all possible combinations of different values of means and standard deviations. The two most commonly provided sets of tables are (i) the area under the frequency distribution curve, and (ii) the so-called percentage points.

Table for area under the curve of the normal distribution

The table for the area under the frequency distribution curve of the normal distribution is useful for determining the proportion of the population which has values in some specified range. This will be illustrated for the distribution shown in Figures 4.1 and 4.2 of the heights of adult men in the United Kingdom, which is approximately normal with mean $\mu = 171.5$ cm and standard deviation $\sigma = 6.5$ cm.

Area in upper tail of distribution

The normal distribution can be used to estimate, for example, the proportion of men taller than 180 cm. This proportion is represented by the fraction of the area under the frequency distribution curve that is above 180 cm. The corresponding SND is:

$$z = \frac{180 - 171.5}{6.5} = 1.31$$

This is equivalent to the proportion of the area of the standard normal distribution that is above 1.31. This area is illustrated in Figure 4.3(a) and can be found from Table A1. The rows of the table refer to z to one decimal place and the columns to the second decimal place. Thus the area above 1.31 is

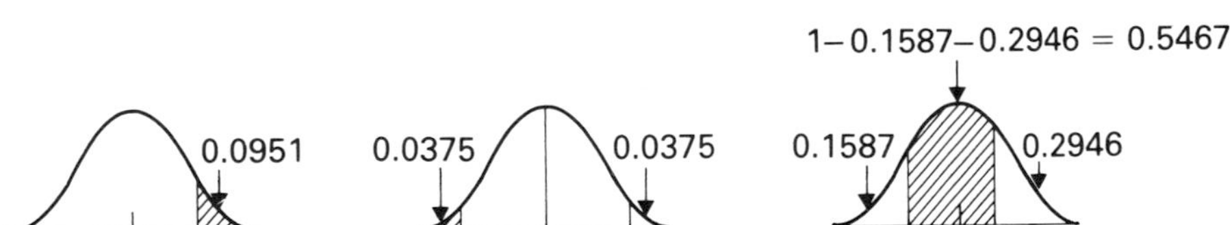

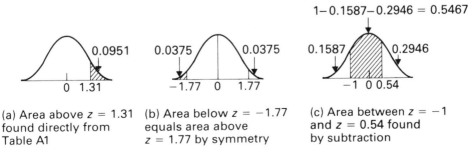

(a) Area above $z = 1.31$ found directly from Table A1

(b) Area below $z = -1.77$ equals area above $z = 1.77$ by symmetry

(c) Area between $z = -1$ and $z = 0.54$ found by subtraction

Figure 4.3 Examples of the calculation of areas of the standard normal distribution.

given in row 1.3 and column 0.01 and is 0.0951. We conclude that a fraction 0.0951, or equivalently 9.51%, of adult men are taller than 180 cm.

Area in lower tail of distribution

The proportion of men shorter than 160 cm, for example, can be similarly estimated.

$$z = \frac{160 - 171.5}{6.5} = -1.77$$

The required area is illustrated in Figure 4.3(b). As the standard normal distribution is symmetrical about zero the area below $z = -1.77$ is equal to the area above $z = 1.77$ and is 0.0375. Thus 3.75% of men are shorter than 160 cm.

Area of distribution between two values

The proportion of men with a height between, for example, 165 cm and 175 cm is estimated by finding the proportions of men shorter than 165 cm and taller than 175 cm and subtracting these from 1. This is illustrated in Figure 4.3(c).

(i) SND corresponding to 165 cm is:

$$z = \frac{165 - 171.5}{6.5} = -1$$

Proportion below this height is 0.1587.

(ii) SND corresponding to 175 cm is:

$$z = \frac{175 - 171.5}{6.5} = 0.54$$

Proportion above this height is 0.2946.

(iii) Proportion of men with heights between 165 cm and 175 cm
$= 1 -$ proportion below 165 cm $-$ proportion above 175 cm
$= 1 - 0.1587 - 0.2946 = 0.5467$ or 54.67%

Value corresponding to specified tail area

Table A1 can also be used the other way round, that is starting with an area and finding the corresponding z value. For example, what height is exceeded by 5% or 0.05 of the population? Looking through the table the closest value to 0.05 is found in row 1.6 and column 0.04 and so the required z value is 1.64. The corresponding height is found by inverting the definition of SND to give:

$$x = \mu + z\sigma$$

and is $171.5 + 1.64 \times 6.5 = 182.2$ cm.

Percentage points of the normal distribution

An interpretation of the SND that is sometimes useful is that it expresses the value of the variable in terms of the number of standard deviations it is away from the mean. This is shown on the scale of the original variable in Figure 4.4. Thus, for example, $z = 1$ corresponds to a value which is one standard deviation above the mean and $z = -1$ to one standard deviation below the mean. The areas above $z = 1$ and below $z = -1$ are both 0.1587 or 15.87%. Therefore 31.74% (2 × 15.87%) of the distribution is further than one standard deviation from the mean, or equivalently 68.26% of the distribution lies within one standard deviation of the mean. Similarly, 4.55% of the distribution is further than two standard deviations from the mean, or equivalently 95.45% of the distribution lies within two standard deviations of the mean. This is the justification for the practical interpretation of the standard deviation given in Chapter 3.

The z value encompassing exactly 95% of the distribution between $-z$ and z is 1.96 (Figure 4.5a). 1.96 is said to be the 5% **percentage point** of the normal distribution, as 5% of the distribution is further than 1.96 standard deviations from the mean ($2\frac{1}{2}$% in each tail). Similarly, 2.58 is the 1%

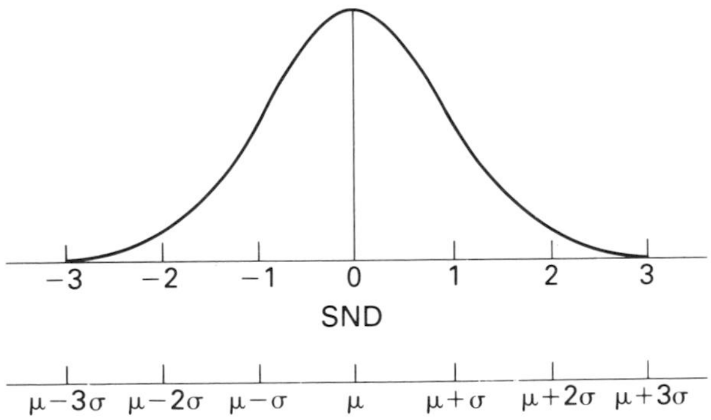

Figure 4.4 Interpretation of SND in terms of a scale showing the number of standard deviations from the mean.

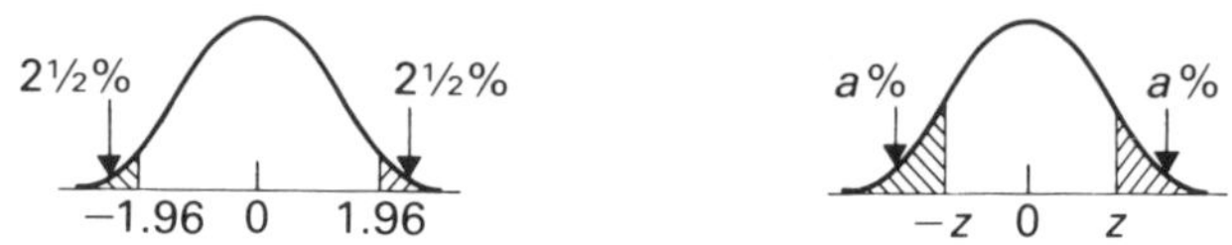

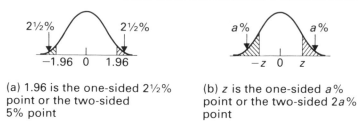

(a) 1.96 is the one-sided 2½% point or the two-sided 5% point

(b) z is the one-sided a% point or the two-sided $2a$% point

Figure 4.5 Percentage points of the normal distribution.

percentage point. The commonly used percentage points are tabulated in Table A2. Note that they could also be found from Table A1 in the way described above.

The percentage points described here are known as **two-sided** percentage points, as they cover extreme observations in both the upper and lower tails of the distribution. Some books tabulate **one-sided** percentage points, referring to just one tail of the distribution. The one-sided a% point is the same as the two-sided $2a$% point (Figure 4.5b). For example, 1.96 is the one-sided $2\frac{1}{2}$% point, as $2\frac{1}{2}$% of the standard normal distribution is above 1.96 (or equivalently $2\frac{1}{2}$% is below -1.96) and it is the two-sided 5% point. This difference is discussed again in Chapter 6 in the context of significance testing.

CHAPTER 5

Confidence Interval for a Mean

Introduction

Sampling variation and the standard error of a sample mean were discussed in Chapter 3. We now consider how we can use the sample mean and its standard error to tell us about the likely values of the population mean, which is usually unknown.

Large sample case (normal distribution)

It was noted in Chapter 3 that approximately 95% of the sample means in the distribution obtained by repeated sampling would lie within two standard errors above or below the population mean. This was based on assuming a normal distribution for the sample means, of which the mean is the population mean, μ, and the standard deviation is the standard error of the sample means, $\sigma/\sqrt{n}$. This is justified where the sample is large, say n greater than 60, since it is nearly always the case that the distribution of sample means *is* normal (*see below*); furthermore, the sample standard deviation, s, is a reliable estimate of the population standard deviation, σ, which is usually not known. From Chapter 4 we can therefore state a little more precisely that 95% of the sample means should lie within 1.96 standard errors above or below the population mean, 1.96 being the 5% point of the standard normal distribution. There is therefore a 95% probability that a particular sample mean lies within 1.96 standard errors above or below the population mean.

In practice, this result is used to estimate from the observed sample mean ($\bar{x}$) and its standard error (s.e. $= s/\sqrt{n}$) a range within which the population mean is likely to lie. As there is a 95% probability that the sample mean lies within 1.96 standard errors above or below the population mean, there is a 95% probability that the interval between $\bar{x} - 1.96$ s.e. and $\bar{x} + 1.96$ s.e. contains the (unknown) population mean. The interval from $\bar{x} - 1.96$ s.e. to $\bar{x} + 1.96$ s.e. therefore represents likely values for the population mean. It is called the 95% **confidence interval** (c.i.) for the population mean, and $\bar{x} + 1.96$ s.e. and $\bar{x} - 1.96$ s.e. are the upper and lower 95% **confidence limits** for the population mean, respectively.

Large-sample 95% c.i. $= \bar{x} \pm (1.96 \times s/\sqrt{n})$

Confidence intervals for percentages other than 95% are calculated in the same way using the appropriate percentage point, z', of the standard normal distribution in place of 1.96. For example, the 99% confidence interval is $\bar{x} \pm (2.58 \times \text{s.e.})$

$$\text{Large-sample c.i.} = \bar{x} \pm (z' \times s/\sqrt{n})$$

Example 5.1

As part of a malaria control programme it was planned to spray all the 10 000 houses in a rural area with insecticide and it was necessary to estimate the amount that would be required. Since it was not feasible to measure all 10 000 houses, a random sample of 100 houses was chosen and the sprayable surface of each of these was measured.

The mean sprayable surface area for these 100 houses was 23.2 m^2 and the standard deviation was 5.9 m^2. It is unlikely that the mean surface area of this sample of 100 houses ($\bar{x}$) exactly equals the mean surface area of all 10 000 houses (μ). Its precision is measured by the standard error $\sigma/\sqrt{n}$, estimated by $s/\sqrt{n} = 5.9/\sqrt{100} = 0.6\ m^2$. There is a 95% probability that the sample mean of 23.2 m^2 differs from the population mean by less than 1.96 s.e. $= 1.96 \times 0.6 = 1.2\ m^2$. The 95% confidence interval is:

$$\bar{x} \pm 1.96s/\sqrt{n} = 23.2 \pm 1.2 = 22.0 \text{ to } 24.4\ m^2$$

It was decided to use the upper 95% confidence limit in budgeting for the amount of insecticide required as it was preferable to overestimate rather than underestimate the amount. One litre of insecticide is sufficient to spray 50 m^2 and so the amount budgeted for was:

$$10\,000 \times 24.4/50 = 4880 \text{ litres}$$

There is still a possibility, however, that this is too little insecticide. The interval 22.0–44.4 m^2 gives the likely range of values for the mean surface area of all 10 000 houses. There is a 95% probability that this interval contains the population mean *but* a 5% probability that it does not, with a $2\frac{1}{2}$% probability ($\frac{1}{2} \times 5\%$) that the estimate based on the upper confidence limit is too small. A more cautious estimate for the amount of insecticide required would be based on a wider confidence interval, such as 99%, giving a smaller probability ($\frac{1}{2}$%) that too little would be estimated.

Smaller samples

In the calculation of confidence intervals so far described the sample size has been assumed to be large (greater than 60). When the sample size is not large, two aspects may alter. Firstly, the sample standard deviation, s, which is itself subject to sampling variation, may not be a reliable estimate for σ. Secondly, when the distribution in the population is not normal, the distribution of the sample mean may also be non-normal.

The second of these effects is of practical importance only when the sample size is very small (less than say 15) *and* when the distribution in the population is extremely non-normal. This is because of a remarkable and very useful mathematical property known as the **central limit theorem**, which states that even when a variable is not normally distributed the sample mean will tend to be normally distributed. (A practical demonstration of this property can easily be had by carrying out a sampling game like Example 3.4, but with the 250 blood pressures replaced by a non-normally distributed population.) The larger the sample the closer the sample mean is to being normally distributed; the number needed to give a close approximation to normality depends on how non-normal the population is, but in most circumstances a sample size of 15 or more is enough.

Because of the central limit theorem, it is usually only the first of the above points, namely the sampling variation in s, that invalidates the use of the normal distribution in the calculation of confidence intervals. Instead a distribution called the t distribution is used. Strictly speaking, this is valid only if the *population* is normally distributed. The use of the t distribution has been shown to be justified, however, except where the population is extremely non-normal. (This property is called **robustness**.) What to do in cases of severe non-normality is described later.

Confidence interval using t *distribution*

The earlier calculation of a confidence interval using the normal distribution was based on the fact that $(\bar{x}-\mu)/(\sigma/\sqrt{n})$ is a value from the standard normal distribution, and that for large samples we could use s in place of σ. In fact, $(\bar{x}-\mu)/(s/\sqrt{n})$ is a value not from the standard normal distribution but from a distribution called the **t distribution with $(n-1)$ degrees of freedom**. This distribution was introduced by W. S. Gossett, who used the pen-name 'Student', and is often called Student's t distribution. Like the normal distribution, the t distribution is a symmetrical bell-shaped distribution with a mean of zero, but it is more spread out, having longer tails (Figure 5.1).

The exact shape of the t distribution depends on the degrees of freedom (d.f.), $n-1$, of the sample standard deviation s; the fewer the degrees of freedom, the more the t distribution is spread out. The percentage points are tabulated for various degrees of freedom in Table A3. For example, if the sample size is 8, the degrees of freedom are 7 and the 5% point is 2.36. In this

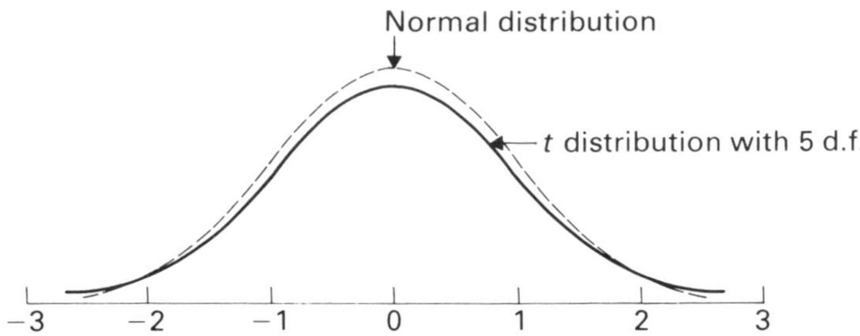

Figure 5.1 t distribution with 5 degrees of freedom compared to the normal distribution.

case the 95% confidence interval using the sample standard deviation s would be $x \pm 2.36\, s/\sqrt{n}$. In general a confidence interval is calculated using t', the appropriate percentage point of the t distribution with $(n-1)$ degrees of freedom.

$$\text{Small-sample c.i.} = \bar{x} \pm (t' \times s/\sqrt{n})$$

For small degrees of freedom the percentage points of the t distribution are appreciably larger in value than the corresponding percentage points of the normal distribution. This is because the sample standard deviation s may be a poor estimate of the population value σ, and when this uncertainty is taken into account the resulting confidence interval is considerably wider than if σ were reliably known. For large degrees of freedom the t distribution is almost the same as the standard normal distribution, since s is a good estimate of σ. The bottom row of Table A3 gives the percentage points for the t distribution with an infinite number (∞) of degrees of freedom and it may be seen by comparison with Table A2 that these are the same as for the normal distribution.

Example 5.2

The following are the numbers of hours of relief obtained by six arthritic patients after receiving a new drug:

2.2, 2.4, 4.9, 2.5, 3.7, 4.3 hours

$\bar{x} = 3.3$ hours, $s = 1.13$ hours, $n = 6$, d.f. $= n - 1 = 5$

$s/\sqrt{n} = 0.46$ hours

The 5% point of the t distribution with 5 degrees of freedom is 2.57, and so the 95% confidence interval for the average number of hours of relief for arthritic patients in general is:

$$3.3 \pm 2.57 \times 0.46 = 3.3 \pm 1.2 = 2.1 \text{ to } 4.5 \text{ hours}$$

Severe non-normality

When the distribution in the population is markedly non-normal, it may be desirable to transform the scale on which the variable x is measured so as to make its distribution on the new scale more normal (*see* Chapter 19). An alternative is to calculate a **non-parametric** confidence interval (Chapter 20), although this procedure is complicated.

Summary of alternatives

Table 5.1 summarizes which procedure to use in constructing a confidence interval. There is no precise boundary between approximate normality and non-normality but, for example, a reverse J-shaped distribution (Figure 2.6b) is severely non-normal, and a skewed distribution (Figure 2.5b or c) is moderately non-normal.

Table 5.1 Recommended procedures for constructing a confidence interval.

(a) Population standard deviation σ unknown.

	Population distribution	
Sample size	Approximately normal	Severely non-normal*
60 or more	$\bar{x} \pm (z' \times s/\sqrt{n})$	$\bar{x} \pm (z' \times s/\sqrt{n})$
Less than 60	$\bar{x} \pm (t' \times s/\sqrt{n})$	Non-parametric

(b) Population standard deviation σ known.

	Population distribution	
Sample size	Approximately normal	Severely non-normal*
15 or more	$\bar{x} \pm (z' \times \sigma/\sqrt{n})$	$\bar{x} \pm (z' \times \sigma/\sqrt{n})$
Less than 15	$\bar{x} \pm (z' \times \sigma/\sqrt{n})$	Non-parametric

* It is preferable to transform the scale of measurement to make the distribution more normal (*see* Chapter 19).

In rare instances the population standard deviation, σ, is known and therefore not estimated from the sample. When this occurs the standard normal distribution percentage points are used to give the confidence interval regardless of sample size, provided the population distribution is not severely non-normal (in which case see the preceding paragraph).

CHAPTER 6

Significance Tests for a Single Mean

Introduction

In Chapter 5 we discussed how a sample mean and its standard error are used to construct a confidence interval representing the likely values for the population mean. In this chapter we describe the opposite but related approach of asking whether the sample mean is consistent with a certain hypothesized value for the population mean. The method for assessing this is known as significance testing. It is usually based on either the t distribution or the normal distribution, the factors governing the choice being exactly the same as those for confidence intervals. A particular but common form of the one-sample t test, the paired t test, will be described first. This will be followed by the general form of the one-sample t test and finally by the one-sample normal test.

Paired t test

The paired t test is used to test whether the difference between a pair of variables measured on each individual is, on average, zero. It is most easily described in relation to a particular example. Consider the results of a clinical trial to test the effectiveness of a sleeping drug in which the sleep of 10 patients was observed during one night with the drug and one night with a placebo. The results obtained are shown in Table 6.1. For each patient a pair of sleep times, namely those with the drug and with the placebo, was recorded and the difference between these calculated. The average number of additional hours slept with the drug compared with the placebo was $\bar{x} = 1.78$, and the standard deviation was $s = 1.77$ hours. The standard error is $s/\sqrt{n} = 1.77/\sqrt{10} = 0.56$ hours.

Even if the drug had no effect the average sleep times with the drug and with the placebo would be very unlikely to have been exactly the same. There are therefore two possible explanations for the observed increase. The first is that it was simply due to chance variation and that in general the drug and placebo give the same amount of sleep. The second explanation is that the observed increase in sleep time was due to a real effect of the drug. A **significance test** is used to decide which is the more likely explanation.

Table 6.1 Results of a placebo-controlled clinical trial to test the effectiveness of a sleeping drug.

	Hours of sleep		
Patient	Drug	Placebo	Difference
1	6.1	5.2	0.9
2	7.0	7.9	−0.9
3	8.2	3.9	4.3
4	7.6	4.7	2.9
5	6.5	5.3	1.2
6	8.4	5.4	3.0
7	6.9	4.2	2.7
8	6.7	6.1	0.6
9	7.4	3.8	3.6
10	5.8	6.3	−0.5
Mean	7.06	5.28	1.78

The test begins by hypothesizing that the first explanation (chance) is true. The first step is thus to define the **null hypothesis** which asserts that there is no real difference in sleep time with the drug or the placebo, or in other words that the true mean difference (μ) is zero. The next step is to calculate the likelihood that, if the null hypothesis were true, the observed value ($\bar{x}$) could just be due to chance variation. This is done by working out the probability of getting a difference in sleep times as large as or larger than the one observed. This probability is called the **significance level** of the result. The idea is to abandon the null hypothesis, that is reject the first explanation (chance) in favour of the second (real effect), only if this probability is very small.

We use the t distribution, and in particular its percentage points, to calculate the significance level of the result. From Chapter 5 we know that, provided the difference in hours slept is normally distributed, $(\bar{x}-\mu)/(s/\sqrt{n})$ is a value from the t distribution with 9 degrees of freedom. The null hypothesis of an average difference in sleep time of zero is equivalent to the population mean, μ, being zero and so:

$$\text{Paired } t = \frac{\bar{x}}{s/\sqrt{n}}, \quad \text{d.f.} = n-1$$

The larger the size of t, the less likely it is that the result is due to chance. (The sign of the t value is ignored.) In this example the t value corresponding to a difference in sleep time of 1.78 hours is:

$$t = 1.78/0.56 = 3.18, \quad \text{d.f.} = 9$$

The (two-sided) 5% percentage point of the t distribution with 9 degrees of freedom is 2.26 (Table A3), which means that there is a 5% probability of a t value larger in size than 2.26. The 2% percentage point is 2.82 and the 1% percentage point is 3.25. The observed t value of 3.18 is between 2.82 and 3.25. Its associated probability is therefore between 2% and 1% (Figure 6.1). The difference in sleep times is said to be **significant at the 2% level**, as the probability that such a large difference could be due to chance is less than 2%. This is often written $P < 0.02$ with the probability expressed as a decimal fraction rather than as a percentage. Since this probability is small, it is concluded that the null hypothesis is implausible and that the trial suggests that the drug does affect sleep time.

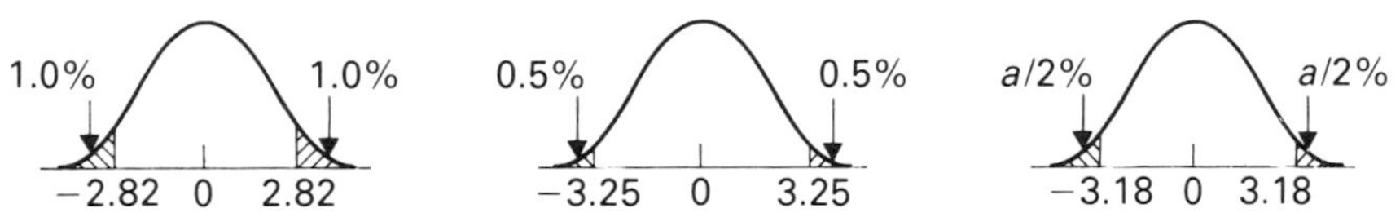

(a) 2.82 is the 2% point

(b) 3.25 is the 1% point

(c) 3.18 is between 2.82 and 3.25 and so the total shaded area (a%) is between 2% and 1%

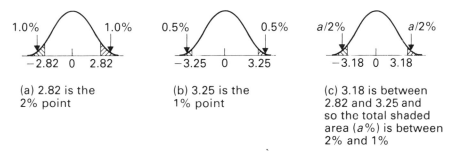

Figure 6.1 The significance of a value of 3.18 from the t distribution with 9 degrees of freedom.

The *smaller* the significance level the *more* significant a result is said to be, since it furnishes stronger evidence against the null hypothesis. It is common practice to consider a probability smaller than 5% as reasonable evidence against the null hypothesis, a probability smaller than 1% as strong evidence against it, and one smaller than 0.1% as very strong evidence in favour of a real effect. A probability greater than 5% is said to be non-significant as it is usually thought that such a result shows reasonable consistency with the null hypothesis. This does not mean that the null hypothesis is necessarily true, however, only that there is no strong evidence against it.

In theory it would be possible to calculate the *exact* probability corresponding to a t value of 3.18, and some computer packages do give this. To do this by hand, however, would require a detailed table (similar to Table A1 for the normal distribution) for each value of the degrees of freedom for the t distribution. For most purposes it is sufficient simply to compare the t value with the percentage points for the appropriate degrees of freedom.

Having established that the drug appears to have a real effect we should say something more about how much extra sleep it would be estimated to give in general. We do this by calculating, for example, the 95% confidence interval. This is $1.78 \pm (2.26 \times 0.56)$ which is 0.51 to 3.05 hours.

Relationship between confidence intervals and significance tests

There is a very close link between confidence interval estimation and significance testing. The confidence interval gives the range of values for the (unknown) population mean that are consistent with the data, while the significance test assesses whether the data are consistent with one particular hypothesized value. Thus, if a result is significantly different from the hypothesized value at a chosen significance level, the corresponding confidence interval will not include this value. On the other hand, if the result is not significant, the confidence interval will include the hypothesized value. In the above example, the observed sample mean (1.78 additional hours slept with the drug) was significantly different from zero at the 5% level, and zero was not included in the 95% confidence interval for the population mean. On the other hand, the sample mean was not significantly different from zero at the 1% level, and the 99% confidence interval ($1.78 \pm 3.25 \times 0.56 = -0.04$ to 3.60 hours) for the population mean does include the value zero.

One-sided and two-sided significance tests

The significance test described above was **two-sided**, since departures from the null hypothesis in either direction were allowed for. We were concerned only with the size of the t value; its sign was ignored. The null hypothesis was that there was no difference between the drug and placebo, and the alternatives of a difference in either direction (the drug giving more or less sleep than the placebo) were considered possible and of interest. The probabilities of both extremes were included in the calculation of the significance level; the two-sided percentage points of the t distribution were used.

A **one-sided** test would have been appropriate if it had been considered that the drug could give either more or the same amount of sleep as the placebo, but could not give less. If this were the case, a result showing that the drug gave on average less sleep would automatically be attributed to chance variation rather than to any real effect, however big the observed reduction in the mean hours of sleep. The significance test would be based only on the upper tail of the t distribution and one-sided percentage points would be used. In this example the drug gave an average of 1.78 hours more sleep and the t value was 3.18 with 9 degrees of freedom. This exceeds the one-sided 1%

point, 2.82, and so using a one-sided test this is significant at the 1% level. (Note that 2.82 is the usual two-sided 2% point, and recall that the two-sided test was significant at the 2% but not the 1% level.)

Two-sided tests are appropriate in the great majority of cases. A one-sided test may be tempting as it is more likely to give a significant result but, for this reason, it also runs a greater risk of inappropriately rejecting the null hypothesis and falsely concluding that there is a real effect. A one-sided test should be used only when there are clear reasons for doing so. This should be decided *before* the data are collected, not after, and should be clearly stated when the results are presented.

One-sample *t* test

The paired t test is a special case of the one-sample t test which tests whether a sample mean is different from some specified value, μ, which need not be zero. The general formula is:

$$t = \frac{\bar{x} - \mu}{s/\sqrt{n}}, \quad \text{d.f.} = n - 1$$

Example 6.1

The following are the heights in centimetres of 24 two-year-old Jamaican boys with homozygous sickle cell disease (SS).

84.4	89.9	89.0	81.9	87.0	78.5	84.1	86.3
80.6	80.0	81.3	86.8	83.4	89.8	85.4	80.6
85.0	82.5	80.7	84.3	85.4	85.0	85.5	81.9

Height and weight standards for the United Kingdom give a reference height for two-year-old males of 86.5 cm. Does the above sample suggest that two-year-old male SS children differ in height from the standards?

$$\bar{x} = 84.1 \text{ cm}, \quad s = 3.11 \text{ cm}, \quad n = 24, \quad s/\sqrt{n} = 0.63 \text{ cm}$$

The null hypothesis is that the mean height of two-year-old male SS children is 86.5 cm.

$$t = \frac{\bar{x} - 86.5}{s/\sqrt{n}} = \frac{84.1 - 86.5}{0.63} = -3.81, \quad \text{d.f.} = 23, \ P < 0.001$$

Thus the mean height of the sample of Jamaican male SS children is significantly lower than the height given in the standards for the United Kingdom ($P < 0.001$). Note that care is needed in interpreting this result since the growth of Jamaican SS children has been compared with standards compiled for the United Kingdom, and not for healthy Jamaican children. It may well be that sickle cell disease leads to stunting of growth, but a comparison with Jamaican children without the disease would be needed to demonstrate this. Methods for comparing the means from two samples are described in Chapter 7.

Normal test

As in the case of confidence interval estimation, when testing the mean of a large sample (size 60 or more), or on the rare occasions when the population standard deviation is known, the normal rather than the t distribution is used. The form of the significance test is exactly the same.

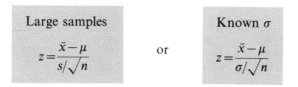

Large samples

$$z = \frac{\bar{x} - \mu}{s/\sqrt{n}}$$

or

Known σ

$$z = \frac{\bar{x} - \mu}{\sigma/\sqrt{n}}$$

There seems to be no generally accepted name for this test. It is sometimes called the normal test, sometimes the z test, and sometimes the SND (standard normal deviate) test. The first of these names will be used in this book.

Types of error in significance testing

As has been described, significance testing is a method for assessing whether a result is likely to be due to chance or to some real effect. It cannot *prove* that it is one or the other and one of two types of errors may occur in its use. The null hypothesis may be rejected when it is in fact true, or alternatively we may fail to reject it when it is false. These are called type I and type II errors respectively (Table 6.2).

Table 6.2 Types of error in significance testing.

	Reality	
Conclusion of significance test	Null hypothesis is true	Null hypothesis is false
Reject null hypothesis	Type I error (probability = significance)	Correct conclusion (probability = power)
Do not reject null hypothesis	Correct conclusion (probability = 1 − significance)	Type II error (probability = 1 − power)

Recall that the significance level of a test equals the probability of occurrence of a result as extreme as or more extreme than that observed, if the null hypothesis were true. The probability that we commit a type I error and wrongly reject the null hypothesis therefore equals the significance level of the test. For example, there is a 5% probability that sampling variation alone will lead to a result significant at the 5% level, and so if we judge such a result as evidence against the null hypothesis, there is a 5% probability that we are making an error in doing so (Figure 6.2a).

The second type of error is that the null hypothesis is not rejected when it is false. This occurs because of overlap between the real sampling distribution of the sample mean about the population mean, $\mu'(\neq \mu)$, and the acceptance

(a)

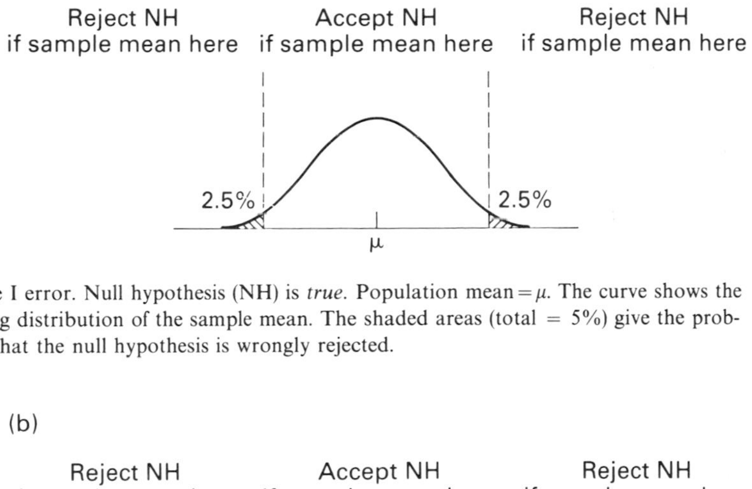

(a) Type I error. Null hypothesis (NH) is *true*. Population mean $= \mu$. The curve shows the sampling distribution of the sample mean. The shaded areas (total = 5%) give the probability that the null hypothesis is wrongly rejected.

(b)

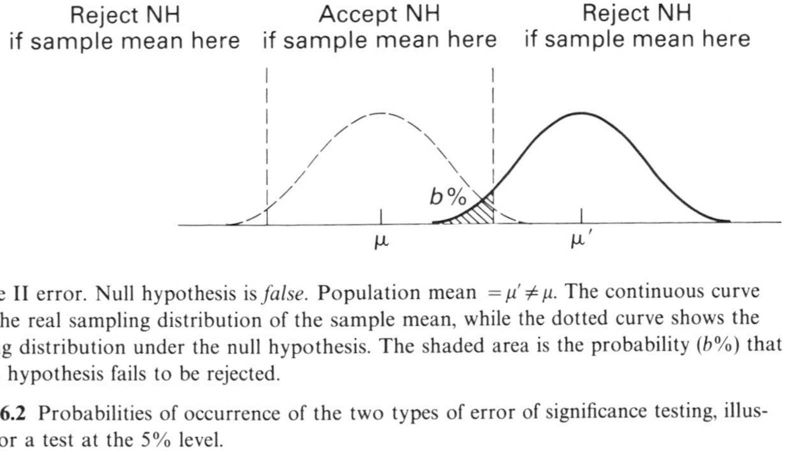

(b) Type II error. Null hypothesis is *false*. Population mean $= \mu' \neq \mu$. The continuous curve shows the real sampling distribution of the sample mean, while the dotted curve shows the sampling distribution under the null hypothesis. The shaded area is the probability (b%) that the null hypothesis fails to be rejected.

Figure 6.2 Probabilities of occurrence of the two types of error of significance testing, illustrated for a test at the 5% level.

region for the null hypothesis based on the hypothesized sampling distribution about the incorrect mean, μ. This is illustrated in Figure 6.2(b). The shaded area shows the proportion (b%) of the real sampling distribution that would fall within the acceptance region for the null hypothesis, i.e. that would appear consistent with the null hypothesis at the 5% level. If a lower significance level were used, making the probability of a type I error smaller, the size of the shaded area would be increased, leading to a larger probability of failing to reject the null hypothesis. The converse is also true. The probability that we do not make a type II error ($100 - b$%) is called the **power** of the test. This is discussed in more detail in the context of sample size determination in Chapter 26. In brief, increasing the sample size increases the power, since the sampling distribution curves in Figure 6.2(b) would be taller and narrower and therefore overlap less.

CHAPTER 7

Comparison of Two Means

Introduction

The use of the t and normal tests to compare a single sample mean with a hypothesized value of the population mean was discussed in Chapter 6. In this chapter we describe the use of these tests in comparing the means from two different samples, for example the mean birth weights of children born to heavy smokers and of children born to non-smokers. The rules for which of the tests to use are similar to those for the one-sample case, and the form of the tests is the same, namely the quantity to be tested divided by its standard error. Unlike the one-sample case, however, the formulae for the t and normal tests are different. This is because the calculations of the standard errors are different, since the t test requires an extra assumption, namely that the two population standard deviations are equal. Details are given below. Confidence intervals are calculated in the usual way.

It should be noted that these two-sample tests are not appropriate for comparing the means of two variables measured on the *same sample*. In this case the difference between each *pair* of observations should be calculated and the one-sample paired test used, as described in Chapter 6.

Sampling distribution of difference between two means

The difference, $\bar{x}_1 - \bar{x}_2$, between the means of two independent samples is normally distributed provided that each of the means is normally distributed. The mean of this distribution is simply the difference between the two population means, $\mu_1 - \mu_2$. The null hypothesis for the significance test is that these means are equal, that is $\mu_1 - \mu_2 = 0$. The formula for the standard error is based on a combination of the standard errors of the individual means.

$$\text{s.e.} = \sqrt{(\sigma_1^2/n_1 + \sigma_2^2/n_2)}$$

This is estimated from the samples using the sample standard deviations, s_1 and s_2.

Normal test (large samples or known standard deviations)

The normal test is used when both the samples are large or in the rare instances when the population standard deviations are known.

Large samples		Known σ's
$z=\dfrac{\bar{x}_1-\bar{x}_2}{\sqrt{(s_1^2/n_1+s_2^2/n_2)}}$	or	$z=\dfrac{\bar{x}_1-\bar{x}_2}{\sqrt{(\sigma_1^2/n_1+\sigma_2^2/n_2)}}$

Consider the following results from a malaria screening programme in which blood slides from 150 children aged between one and four years were examined for *Plasmodium falciparum* parasites. Parasites were found in 70 of the slides, and the mean haemoglobin level for these children was 10.6 g/100 ml with standard deviation 1.4 g/100 ml. The mean haemoglobin level for the other 80 children was 11.5 g/100 ml with standard deviation 1.3 g/100 ml. Does this suggest that haemoglobin level is lowered during infection with *P. falciparum*? As both the samples are large the normal test can be used.

$$n_1=70,\quad \bar{x}_1=10.6,\quad s_1=1.4$$
$$n_2=80,\quad \bar{x}_2=11.5,\quad s_2=1.3$$

$$z=\frac{10.6-11.5}{\sqrt{(1.4^2/70+1.3^2/80)}}=\frac{-0.9}{0.2216}=-4.06,\ P<0.001$$

This result is significant at the 0.1% level since 4.06 is larger than 3.29, the 0.1% percentage point of the normal distribution (Table A2). Thus the mean haemoglobin level of the children with *P. falciparum* parasitaemia was significantly lower ($P<0.001$) than that of those without.

Confidence interval

Large samples		Known σ's
c.i. $=(\bar{x}_1-\bar{x}_2)\pm(z'\times \text{s.e.})$	or	c.i. $=(\bar{x}_1-\bar{x}_2)\pm(z'\times \text{s.e.})$
s.e. $=\sqrt{(s_1^2/n_1+s_2^2/n_2)}$		s.e. $=\sqrt{(\sigma_1^2/n_1+\sigma_2^2/n_2)}$

The confidence interval is calculated using z', the appropriate percentage point of the normal distribution. The 95% confidence interval for the difference between the mean haemoglobin levels in the above example is:

$$-0.9\pm(1.96\times 0.2216)=-1.33\ \text{to}\ -0.47\ \text{g/100 ml}$$

that is a mean haemoglobin between 0.47 and 1.33 g/100 ml lower in children with parasitaemia.

t test (small samples, equal standard deviations)

The t test is used for small samples. It requires that the population distributions are normal but, as in the one-sample case, is robust against departures from this assumption. When comparing two means, the validity of the t test also depends on the equality of the two population standard deviations. In many situations it is reasonable to assume this equality. If the sample standard deviations are very different in size, however, say if one is twice the other or more, an alternative must be used. This is discussed below.

The formula for the standard error of the difference between the means is simplified to:

$$\text{s.e.} = \sqrt{(\sigma^2/n_1 + \sigma^2/n_2)} \quad \text{or} \quad \sigma\sqrt{(1/n_1 + 1/n_2)}$$

where σ is the common standard deviation. There are two sample estimates of σ from the two samples, s_1 and s_2, and these are combined to give a common estimate, s, of the population standard deviation, with degrees of freedom equal to $(n_1 - 1) + (n_2 - 1) = n_1 + n_2 - 2$.

$$s = \sqrt{\left[\frac{(n_1 - 1)s_1^2 + (n_2 - 1)s_2^2}{(n_1 + n_2 - 2)}\right]}$$

This formula gives greater weight to the estimate from the larger sample as this will be more reliable. The standard error of the difference between the means is estimated by:

$$\text{s.e.} = s\sqrt{(1/n_1 + 1/n_2)}$$

and the t value is calculated as:

$$t = \frac{\bar{x}_1 - \bar{x}_2}{s\sqrt{(1/n_1 + 1/n_2)}}, \quad \text{d.f.} = n_1 + n_2 - 2$$

Table 7.1 shows the birth weights of children born to 15 non-smokers

Table 7.1 Comparison of birth weights of children born to 15 non-smokers with those of children born to 14 heavy smokers.

	Birth weight (kg)	
	Non-smokers	Heavy smokers
	3.99	3.18
	3.79	2.84
	3.60	2.90
	3.73	3.27
	3.21	3.85
	3.60	3.52
	4.08	3.23
	3.61	2.76
	3.83	3.60
	3.31	3.75
	4.13	3.59
	3.26	3.63
	3.54	2.38
	3.51	2.34
	2.71	
$\bar{x}$	3.5933	3.2029
s	0.3707	0.4927
n	15	14

and to 14 heavy smokers. The calculations for the t test to compare these two groups are as follows:

$$s=\sqrt{\left[\frac{(14\times 0.3707^2+13\times 0.4927^2)}{(15+14-2)}\right]}=0.4337 \text{ kg}$$

$$t=\frac{(3.5933-3.2029)}{0.4337\sqrt{(1/15+1/14)}}=\frac{0.3904}{0.1612}=2.42, \text{ d.f.}=15+14-2=27$$

From Table A3 it is seen that 2.42 approximately equals 2.47, the 2% point of the t distribution with 27 degrees of freedom. This result is therefore significant at the 2% level suggesting that on average children born to non-smokers are heavier than children born to heavy smokers.

Confidence interval

$$\text{c.i.} = (\bar{x}_1 - \bar{x}_2) \pm (t' \times \text{s.e.}), \quad \text{s.e.} = s\sqrt{(1/n_1 + 1/n_2)}$$

The confidence interval is calculated using t', the appropriate percentage point of the t distribution with $(n_1 + n_2 - 2)$ degrees of freedom. In the example the 95% confidence interval for the difference between the mean birth weights is:

$$0.3904 \pm (2.05 \times 0.1612) = 0.06 \text{ to } 0.72 \text{ kg}$$

that is between 0.06 and 0.72 kg higher for children born to non-smokers compared with those born to heavy smokers.

Small samples, unequal standard deviations

When the population standard deviations of the two groups are different it is recommended that the first approach should be to seek a suitable change of scale to remedy this (*see* Chapter 19), so that the t test can be used. For example, if the standard deviations seem to be proportional in size to the means, then taking logarithms of the individual values may help. Alternatives are to use a non-parametric test (*see* Chapter 20) or to use either the Fisher–Behrens or the Welch test (Armitage & Berry 1987). Details of the latter tests are not included here as their use is not common.

CHAPTER 8

Comparison of Several Means—Analysis of Variance

Introduction

More complex sets of data comprising more than two groups are common, and their analysis often involves the comparison of the means of the component subgroups. For example, it may be desired to analyse haemoglobin measurements collected as part of a community survey to see how they vary with age and sex, and to see whether any sex difference is the same for all age-groups. Conceivably it would be possible to do this using a series of t tests, comparing the groups two at a time. This is not only practically tedious, however, but theoretically unsound, since carrying out a large number of significance tests is likely to lead to spurious significant results. For example, a significant result at the 5% level would be expected from 5% (one in 20) of all tests performed even if there were no real differences. (See the discussion of type I errors in Chapter 6.)

A completely different approach, called **analysis of variance**, is used instead. The meaning of this name will become obvious later. The methodology is fairly complex. The calculations are time-consuming and are usually carried out using a standard computer package. For these reasons the emphasis in this chapter is on the principles involved, with the aim of giving the reader sufficient knowledge to be able to specify the form of analysis required and to interpret the results. Details of the calculations are included, however, for the simplest case, that of one-way analysis of variance, as these are helpful in understanding the basis of the method and its relationship to the t test.

One-way analysis of variance is appropriate when the subgroups to be compared are defined by just one **factor**, for example in the comparison of means between different socioeconomic classes or between different ethnic groups. Two-way analysis of variance is also described and is appropriate when the subdivision is based on two factors such as age and sex. The methods are easily extended to the comparison of subgroups cross-classified by more than two factors.

A factor is chosen for inclusion in an analysis of variance either because it is desired to compare its different levels or because it represents a source of variation that it is important to take into account. Consider the following example. Following the discovery that coronary heart disease rates differ markedly between different ethnic groups, a survey was carried out to see whether this was reflected in differing mean lipid concentrations for the different ethnic groups. As lipid concentrations are known to vary with age and sex, it is appropriate to include age-group and sex in the analysis of variance as well as ethnic group, although these were not themselves of particular interest in the study. Their inclusion has two benefits. Firstly, the resulting significance test of differences between the ethnic groups is more powerful, that is it is more likely to detect any real differences as being statistically significant. Secondly, it ensures that the ethnic group comparisons are not biased due to different age–sex compositions. (See the discussion of confounding variables in Chapter 14. See also the description of the methods of standardization in Chapter 15, which can be used for the presentation of ethnic group means adjusted for age and sex differences.)

It is also possible to analyse data subdivided by one or more factors using the closely related but more general technique of **multiple regression** which is described in Chapter 10. Both approaches give identical results, but because of its generality multiple regression involves more complicated calculations and is therefore less efficient in these simpler situations. It is recommended, however, that the choice be based on the computer programs available and their relative ease of use.

Some readers may find the content of the rest of this chapter a little difficult. It may be omitted at a first reading.

One-way analysis of variance

One-way analysis of variance is used to compare the means of several groups, for example the mean haemoglobin levels of patients with different types of sickle cell disease (Table 8.1a). The analysis is called one-way as the data are classified just one way, in this case by type of sickle cell disease. The method is based on assessing how much of the overall variation in the data is attributable to differences between the group means, and comparing this with the amount attributable to differences between individuals in the same group. Hence the name analysis of variance.

We start by calculating the variance of all the observations, ignoring their subdivision into groups. Recall from Chapter 3 that the variance is the square of the standard deviation and equals the sum of squared deviations of the observations about the overall mean, divided by the degrees of freedom. One-way analysis of variance partitions this **sum of squares** (SS) into two distinct components:

(i) The sum of squares due to differences between the group means.

(ii) The sum of squares due to differences between the observations within each group. This is also called the **residual** sum of squares.
The total degrees of freedom are similarly divided. The calculations for the sickle cell data are shown in Table 8.1(b) and the results laid out in an analysis of variance table in Table 8.1(c).

The fourth column of the table gives the amount of variation per degree of freedom, and this is called the **mean square** (MS). The significance test for differences between the groups is based on a comparison of the between-groups and within-groups mean squares. If the observed differences in mean haemoglobin levels for the different types of sickle cell disease were simply due to chance variation, the variation between these group means would be about the same size as the variation between individuals with the same type, while if they were real differences the between-groups variation would be larger. The mean squares are compared using the ***F* test**, sometimes called the **variance-ratio** test.

$$F = \frac{\text{Between-groups MS}}{\text{Within-groups MS}}, \quad \text{d.f.} = \text{d.f.}_{\text{Between-groups}}, \text{d.f.}_{\text{Within-groups}} = (k-1, N-k)$$

where N is the total number of observations and k is the number of groups.

F should be about 1 if there are no real differences between the groups and larger than 1 if there are differences. Under the null hypothesis that the differences are simply due to chance, this ratio follows an ***F* distribution** which, in contrast to most distributions, is specified by a *pair* of degrees of freedom: $(k-1)$ degrees of freedom in the numerator and $(N-k)$ in the denominator. The percentage points of the F distribution are tabulated for various pairs of degrees of freedom in Table A4. The columns of the tables refer to the numerator degrees of freedom and the blocks of rows to the denominator degrees of freedom. Within each block there is a separate line for each percentage level. The percentage points are *one-sided* as the test is based only on extreme levels of F *larger* than one.

In Table 8.1(c), $F = 49.94/1.00 = 49.9$ with degrees of freedom (2, 38). The tables of percentage points have rows for 30 and 40 but not 38 degrees of freedom. We may, however, say that the 0.1% percentage point for $F(2, 38)$ is between 8.77 and 8.25, which are the 0.1% percentage points for $F(2, 30)$ and $F(2, 40)$. Clearly 49.9 is greater than either of these. Thus the steady-state haemoglobin levels differ significantly between patients with different types of sickle cell disease ($P < 0.001$), the mean level being lowest for patients with Hb SS disease, intermediate

Table 8.1 One-way analysis of variance: differences in steady-state haemoglobin levels between patients with different types of sickle cell disease. Data from Anionwu *et al.* (1981) *British Medical Journal*, **282**, 283–6.

(a) Data.

Type of sickle cell disease	No. of patients (n_i)	Haemoglobin (g/dl) Mean ($\bar{x}_i$)	s.d. (s_i)	Individual values (x)
Hb SS	16	8.7125	0.8445	7.2, 7.7, 8.0, 8.1, 8.3, 8.4, 8.4, 8.5, 8.6, 8.7, 9.1, 9.1, 9.1, 9.8, 10.1, 10.3
Hb S/β-thalassaemia	10	10.6300	1.2841	8.1, 9.2, 10.0, 10.4, 10.6, 10.9, 11.1, 11.9, 12.0, 12.1
Hb SC	15	12.3000	0.9419	10.7, 11.3, 11.5, 11.6, 11.7, 11.8, 12.0, 12.1, 12.3, 12.6, 12.6, 13.3, 13.3, 13.8, 13.9

(b) Calculations.

$N = \Sigma n_i = 16 + 10 + 15 = 41$, no. of groups $(k) = 3$

$\Sigma x = 7.2 + 7.7 + \ldots + 13.8 + 13.9 - 430.2$

$\Sigma x^2 = 7.2^2 + 7.7^2 + \ldots + 13.8^2 + 13.9^2 = 4651.80$

Total: $\text{SS} = \Sigma(x - \bar{x})^2 = \Sigma x^2 - (\Sigma x)^2/N = 4651.80 - 430.2^2/41 = 137.85$

d.f. $= N - 1 = 40$

Between groups: $\text{SS} = \Sigma n_i(\bar{x}_i - \bar{x})^2$, more easily calculated as $\Sigma n_i \bar{x}_i^2 - (\Sigma x)^2/N$

$= 16 \times 8.7125^2 + 10 \times 10.6300^2 + 15 \times 12.3000^2 - 430.2^2/41 = 99.89$

d.f. $= k - 1 = 2$

Within groups: $\text{SS} = \Sigma(n_i - 1)s_i^2$

$= 15 \times 0.8445^2 + 9 \times 1.2841^2 + 14 \times 0.9419^2 = 37.96$

d.f. $= N - k = 41 - 3 = 38$

(c) Analysis of variance table.

Source of variation	SS	d.f.	$\text{MS} = \frac{\text{SS}}{\text{d.f.}}$	$F = \frac{\text{Between-groups MS}}{\text{Within-groups MS}}$
Between groups	99.89	2	49.94	49.9, $P < 0.001$
Within groups	37.96	38	1.00	
Total	137.85	40		

for patients with Hb S/β-thalassaemia, and highest for patients with Hb SC disease.

Assumptions

There are two assumptions underlying the F test. The first is that the data are normally distributed. The second is that the population value for the standard deviation between individuals is the same for each group. This is estimated by the square root of the within-groups mean square. Moderate departures from normality may be safely ignored, but the effect of unequal standard deviations may be serious. In the latter case, transforming the data may help (*see* Chapter 19).

Relationship with the two-sample t *test*

One-way analysis of variance is an extension of the two-sample t test. When there are only two groups, it gives exactly the same results as the t test. The F value equals the square of the corresponding t value and the percentage points of the F distribution with $(1, N-2)$ degrees of freedom are the same as the square of those of the t distribution with $N-2$ degrees of freedom.

Two-way analysis of variance

Two-way analysis of variance is used when the data are classified in two ways, for example by age-group and sex. The data are said to have a **balanced design** if there are equal numbers of observations in each group and an **unbalanced design** if there are not. Balanced designs are of two types, **with replication** if there is more than one observation in each group and **without replication** if there is only one. The three designs will be described separately.

Balanced design with replication

Table 8.2 shows the results from an experiment in which five male and five female rats of each of three strains were treated with growth hormone. The aims were to find out whether the strains responded to the treatment to the same extent, and whether there was any sex difference. The measure of response was weight gain after seven days.

These data are classified in two ways, by strain and by sex. The design is balanced with replication because there are five observations in each strain–sex group. Two-way analysis of variance divides the total sum of squares into four components:

Table 8.2 Differences in response to growth hormone for five male and five female rats from three different strains.

(a) Mean weight gains in grams with standard deviations in parentheses ($n = 5$ for each group).

	Strain		
Sex	A	B	C
Male	11.9 (0.9)	12.1 (0.7)	12.2 (0.7)
Female	12.3 (1.1)	11.8 (0.6)	13.1 (0.9)

(b) Two-way analysis of variance: balanced design with replication.

Source of variation	SS	d.f.	MS	$F = \frac{\text{MS effect}}{\text{MS residual}}$
Main effects				
Strain	2.63	2	1.32	1.9, $P > 0.1$
Sex	1.16	1	1.16	1.7, $P > 0.1$
Interaction				
Strain × sex	1.65	2	0.83	1.2, $P > 0.1$
Residual	16.86	24	0.70	
Total	22.30	29		

(i) The sum of squares due to *differences between the strains*. This is said to be the **main effect** of the factor, strain. Its associated degrees of freedom are one less than the number of strains and equal 2.
(ii) The sum of squares due to *differences between the sexes*, that is the main effect of sex. Its degrees of freedom equal 1, one less than the number of sexes.
(iii) The sum of squares due to the **interaction** between strain and sex. An interaction means that the strain differences are not the same for both sexes or, equivalently, that the sex difference is not the same for the three strains. The degrees of freedom equal the product of the degrees of freedom of the two main effects, which is $2 \times 1 = 2$.
(iv) The *residual sum of squares* due to differences between the rats within each strain–sex group. Its degrees of freedom equal 24, the product of the number of strains (3), the number of sexes (2) and one less than the number of observations in each group (4).
The main effects and interaction are tested for significance using the F test to compare their mean squares with the residual mean square, as described for one-way analysis of variance. No significant results were obtained in this experiment.

Balanced design without replication

Five different techniques for estimating length of gestation are compared for 10 women in Table 8.3. There is no residual sum of squares calculated in the analysis of variance, since there is only one observation with each technique for each woman. In such a case, the interaction is *assumed* to be due to chance variation, and its mean square is used as an estimate of the residual mean square for calculating the F values of the main effects. As would be expected, the main effect due to differences between the 10 women in their lengths of gestation was significant. This is not of much interest in its own right, but is an important source of variation to be taken into account when comparing the techniques. The main effect for differences between the five techniques was significant at the 5% level ($F=757.85/202.81=3.74$, d.f. $=[4, 36]$).

Subdivision of sum of squares

It is often desirable to examine the differences contributing to a significant effect in more detail. For example, the date of quickening method gave, on average, considerably higher estimates than the other techniques. It is possible to subdivide the main effect sum of squares for techniques as shown in Table 8.3(c) into:

(i) The sum of squares due to the difference between the date of quickening method and the other techniques. This has 1 degree of freedom.

(ii) The remaining sum of squares with 3 degrees of freedom, representing differences among the other four techniques (LMP, VE, US, DAO).

Each subcomponent is tested using an F test in the usual way. This subdivision showed that the date of quickening method differed significantly ($P<0.001$) from the other techniques, but that there were no significant differences among the other four.

Note that the sum of squares for techniques could have been subdivided in various other ways, and into as many independent components as there are degrees of freedom, in this case four. The subdivisions chosen depend on the comparisons of interest and should preferably be decided on *a priori* grounds before the data are analysed. The subdivision is carried out using the **method of linear contrasts**. The reader is referred to Armitage & Berry (1987) for more detail.

Relationship with one-sample t *test*

The two-way analysis of variance for a balanced design without replication is an extension of the one-sample paired t test, comparing the values of more than two variables measured on each individual. In this case there were five

Table 8.3 Lengths of gestation in days for 10 women, estimated by each of five techniques—last menstrual period (LMP), vaginal examination (VE), date of quickening (DOQ), ultrasound (US) and diamine oxidase (DAO) blood test.

(a) Data.

Subject	LMP	VE	DOQ	US	DAO
1	275	273	288	273	244
2	292	283	284	285	329
3	281	274	298	270	252
4	284	275	271	272	258
5	285	294	307	278	275
6	283	279	301	276	279
7	290	265	298	291	295
8	294	277	295	290	271
9	300	304	293	279	271
10	284	297	352	292	284
Mean	286.8	282.1	298.7	280.6	275.8

(b) Two-way analysis of variance: balanced design without replication (interaction MS used as estimate of residual MS for F test).

Source of variation	SS	d.f.	MS	$F = \frac{\text{MS effect}}{\text{MS interaction}}$
Subjects	4437.6	9	493.07	2.43, $P<0.05$
Techniques	3031.4	4	757.85	3.74, $P<0.05$
Interaction	7301.0	36	202.81	
Total	14770.0	49		

(c) Subdivision of the sum of squares due to techniques.

Source of variation	SS	d.f.	MS	$F = \frac{\text{MS effect}}{\text{MS interaction}}$
DOQ compared to other techniques	2415.1	1	2415.10	11.91, $P<0.001$
Differences between LMP, VE, US and DAO	616.3	3	205.43	1.01, $P>0.1$
Techniques	3031.4	4		

variables, lengths of gestation estimated by five different techniques, for each woman. The two approaches give the same results when just two variables are measured, and the F value equals the square of the t value.

Unbalanced design

Table 8.4(a) summarizes data on hookworm infestation and haemoglobin level, collected as part of a survey on parasitic infestations in East Africa. They are classified by two factors, sex and intensity of hookworm infestation. It can be seen that for each sex, haemoglobin level declines with increasing severity of hookworm infestation, and that for each intensity group, mean haemoglobin is lower for females than for males. The design is not balanced, however, since there are different numbers of persons in each group. This means that it is not possible to disentangle the effects of sex and intensity of hookworm infestation, making the interpretation of these data less straightforward.

Table 8.4 Haemoglobin levels (g/dl) according to intensity of infection with hookworm, for adult males and females.

(a) Data.

Intensity of hookworm infestation	Males			Females		
	No.	Mean Hb	s.d.	No.	Mean Hb	s.d.
Negative	22	12.3	1.8	35	11.1	1.1
Low	20	11.9	1.2	27	10.8	1.3
Medium	17	10.7	1.6	14	9.5	1.9
High	15	9.0	1.4	11	8.6	1.7

(b) Two-way analysis of variance: unbalanced design.

Source of variation	SS	d.f.	MS	$F=\frac{\text{MS effect}}{\text{MS residual}}$
Sex	20.94	1	20.94	9.9, $P<0.01$
Intensity of hookworm adjusting for sex	176.68	3	58.89	27.8, $P<0.001$
Interaction	3.24	3	1.08	0.5, $P>0.1$
Residual	324.28	153	2.12	
Total	525.14	160		

The total sum of squares can *not* be divided into independent components attributable to the two factors, and the analysis of variance table is modified as shown in Table 8.4(b). The sum of squares due to a difference between the sexes is calculated first. Unless the two sexes have similar hookworm distributions, this sum of squares will include some of the variation due to differences in hookworm intensity. The *additional* sum of squares due to hookworm intensity is then calculated. This assesses the relationship between haemoglobin level and intensity of hookworm infestation, with adjustment for any sex differences between the hookworm groups. Both main effects were highly significant, that for sex at the 1% level ($F=9.9$, d.f. $=[1, 153]$) and that for intensity of hookworm infestation, after adjustment for sex, at the 0.1% level ($F=27.8$, d.f. $=[3, 153]$). There was no significant interaction.

Alternatively, the effect of hookworm infestation could be allowed for first in the analysis of variance, in which case it would include some of the variation due to differing haemoglobin levels between males and females. The main effect for sex would then represent any sex difference remaining after adjustment for different distributions of intensity of hookworm infestation between males and females. With an unbalanced design it is often sensible to carry out the analysis using both orders. In this example, however, logical considerations suggest that it is more appropriate to include sex first.

Unbalanced data are common, and unavoidable, in survey investigations. Clinical trials and laboratory experiments should, however, be planned to give a balanced design. This planning may not always succeed as, for example, people may default or move out of the area half-way through a trial, or animals may die during the course of an experiment. The analysis of variance routines of some of the smaller computer packages can only be used for balanced designs or for designs with only a very small proportion of **missing values**; in these cases the multiple regression routine should be used for unbalanced designs (*see* Chapter 10).

Fixed and random effects

Factors can be divided into two types, fixed effects (the more common) and random effects. Factors such as sex, age-group, and type of sickle cell disease are all **fixed effects** since their individual levels have specific values; sex is always male or female. In contrast the individual levels of a **random effect** are not of intrinsic interest, but are a sample of levels representative of a source of variation. For example, consider a study to investigate the variation in sodium and sucrose concentrations of home-prepared oral rehydration solutions, in which 10 persons were each asked to prepare eight solutions. In this case, the 10 persons are of interest only as representatives of the variation between solutions prepared by different persons. Persons is a random effect. In this particular example, as well as testing whether the person effect is significant, we would be interested in estimating the sizes of the variation in concentrations between solutions prepared by the same person, and of the variation between solutions prepared by different persons. These are called **components of variation**. See Huitson (1980) for their method of estimation.

The method of significance testing is the same for fixed and random effects in one-way designs and in two-way designs without replication, but not in two-way designs with replication (or in higher level designs). In the latter, if both effects are fixed, their mean squares are compared with the residual mean square as described above. If, on the other hand, both effects are random, their mean squares are compared with the interaction rather than the residual mean square. If one effect is random and the other fixed, it is the other way round; the random effect mean square is compared with the residual mean square, and the fixed effect mean square with the interaction. These are complex points. The reader interested in a more detailed account should refer to Huitson (1980).

CHAPTER 9

Correlation and Linear Regression

Introduction

Previous chapters have concentrated on the analysis and comparisons of means of a single variable. We now turn to the relationships between different variables and in this chapter look at the closely related techniques of correlation and linear regression for investigating the *linear* association between two continuous variables. Correlation measures the closeness of the association, while linear regression gives the equation of the straight line that best describes it and enables the prediction of one variable from the other.

Correlation

Table 9.1 shows the body weight and plasma volume of eight healthy men. A **scatter diagram** of these data (Figure 9.1) shows that high plasma volume tends to be associated with high weight and vice versa. This association is measured by the **correlation coefficient**, r:

$$r = \frac{\Sigma(x-\bar{x})(y-\bar{y})}{\sqrt{[\Sigma(x-\bar{x})^2\Sigma(y-\bar{y})^2]}}$$

Table 9.1 Plasma volume and body weight in eight healthy men.

Subject	Body weight (kg)	Plasma volume (l)
1	58.0	2.75
2	70.0	2.86
3	74.0	3.37
4	63.5	2.76
5	62.0	2.62
6	70.5	3.49
7	71.0	3.05
8	66.0	3.12

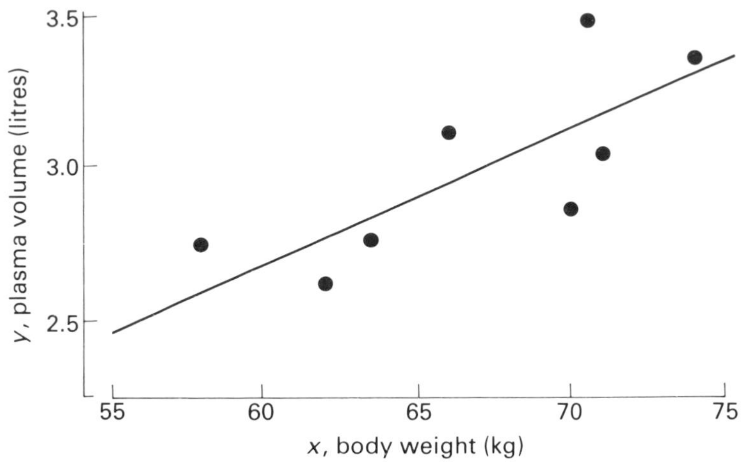

Figure 9.1 Scatter diagram of plasma volume and body weight showing the linear regression line.

where x denotes weight, y denotes plasma volume, and $\bar{x}$ and $\bar{y}$ are the corresponding means. Scatter diagrams illustrating different values of the correlation coefficient are shown in Figure 9.2. The correlation coefficient is always a number between -1 and $+1$, and equals zero if the variables are not associated. It is positive if x and y tend to be high or low together, and the larger its value the closer the association. The maximum value of 1 is obtained if the points in the scatter diagram lie exactly on a straight line. Conversely, the correlation coefficient is negative if high values of y tend to go with low values of x, and vice versa.

It is important to note that a correlation between two variables shows that they are associated but does not necessarily imply a 'cause and effect' relationship. For a fuller discussion see Bradford Hill (1977).

The correlation coefficient is more conveniently calculated by noting:

$$\Sigma(x-\bar{x})(y-\bar{y})=\Sigma xy-(\Sigma x)(\Sigma y)/n$$
$$\Sigma(x-\bar{x})^2=\Sigma x^2-(\Sigma x)^2/n$$
$$\Sigma(y-y)^2=\Sigma y^2-(\Sigma y)^2/n$$

In this example:

$$n=8$$
$$\Sigma x=535 \qquad \bar{x}=66.875 \qquad \Sigma x^2=35983.5$$
$$\Sigma y=24.02 \qquad \bar{y}=3.0025 \qquad \Sigma y^2=72.7980$$
$$\Sigma xy=58.0\times 2.75+70.0\times 2.86\ \ldots\ +66.0\times 3.12=1615.295$$

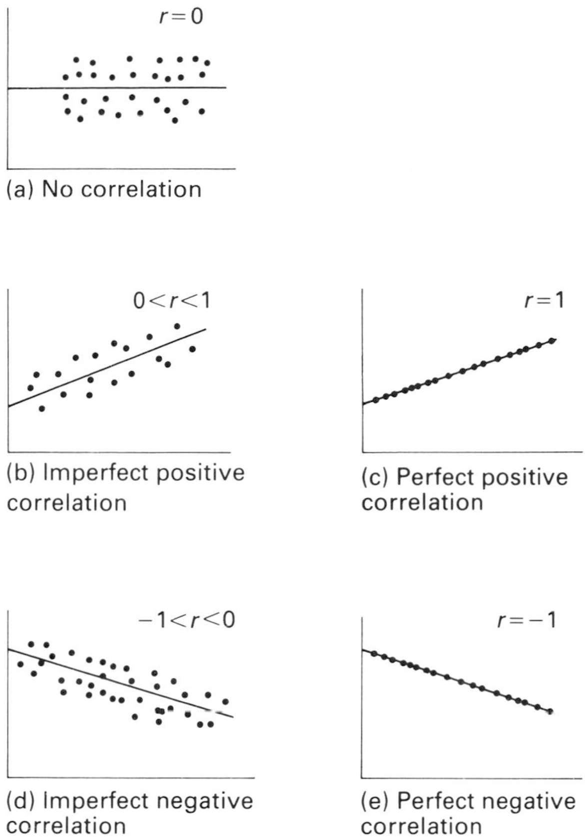

Figure 9.2 Scatter diagrams illustrating different values of the correlation coefficient. Also shown are the regression lines.

therefore:

$$\Sigma(x-\bar{x})(y-\bar{y}) = 1616.295 - 535 \times 24.02/8 = 8.96$$
$$\Sigma(x-\bar{x})^2 = 35983.5 - 535^2/8 = 205.38$$
$$\Sigma(y-\bar{y})^2 = 72.798 - 24.02^2/8 = 0.6780$$

and:

$$r = \frac{8.96}{\sqrt{(205.38 \times 0.6780)}} = 0.76$$

Significance test

A t test is used to test whether r is significantly different from zero, or in other words whether the observed correlation could simply be due to chance.

$$t=r\sqrt{\left[\frac{n-2}{1-r^2}\right]}, \quad \text{d.f.}=n-2$$

In this example:

$$t=0.76\sqrt{\left[\frac{6}{1-0.76^2}\right]}=2.86, \qquad \text{d.f.}=6$$

This is significant at the 5% level, confirming the significance of the apparent association between plasma volume and body weight.

The significance level is a function of both the size of the correlation coefficient and the number of observations. Note that a weak correlation may therefore be statistically significant if based on a large number of observations, while a strong correlation may fail to achieve significance if there are only a few observations.

Linear regression

Linear regression gives the equation of the straight line that describes how the y variable increases (or decreases) with an increase in the x variable. The choice of which variable to call y is important because, unlike for correlation, the two alternatives do not give the same result. y is commonly called the **dependent variable**, and x the **independent**, or **explanatory variable**. In this example, it is obviously the dependence of plasma volume on body weight that is of interest.

The equation of the **regression line** is:

$$y=\mathrm{a}+\mathrm{b}x$$

where a is the **intercept** and b the **slope** of the line (Figure 9.3). The values for a and b are calculated so as to minimize the sum of the squared vertical distances of the points from the line. This is called a **least squares fit** (Figure 9.4). The slope b is sometimes called the **regression coefficient**. It has the same sign as the correlation coefficient. When there is no correlation b equals zero, corresponding to a horizontal regression line at height $\bar{y}$.

$$\mathrm{b}=\frac{\Sigma(x-\bar{x})(y-\bar{y})}{\Sigma(x-\bar{x})^2} \quad \text{and} \quad \mathrm{a}=\bar{y}-\mathrm{b}\bar{x}$$

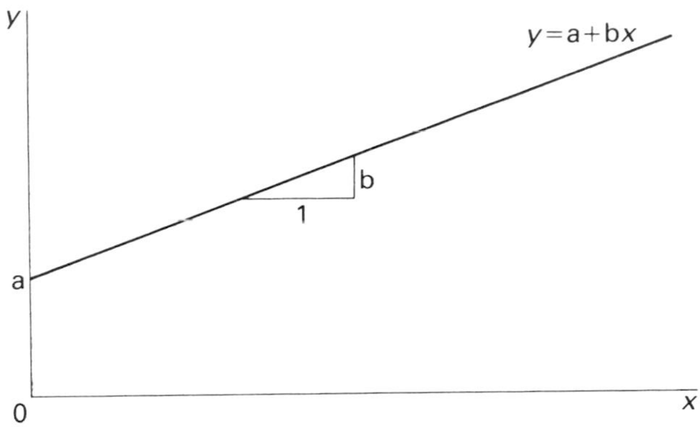

Figure 9.3 The intercept and slope of the regression equation, $y = a + bx$. The intercept, a, is the point where the line crosses the y axis and gives the value of y for $x = 0$. The slope, b, is the increase in y corresponding to a unit increase in x.

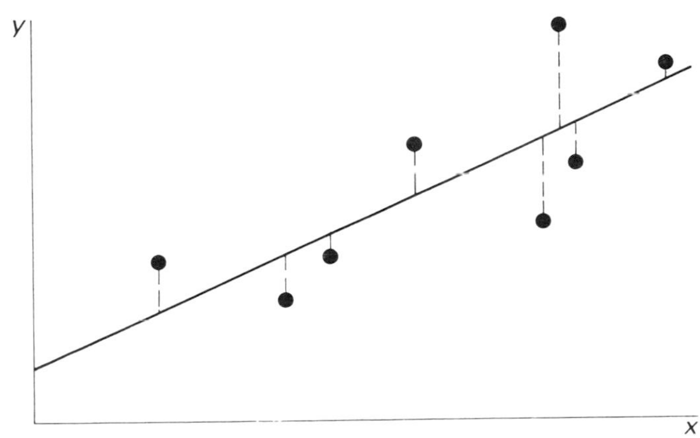

Figure 9.4 Linear regression line, $y = a + bx$, fitted by least squares. a and b are calculated to minimize the sum of squares of the vertical deviations (shown by the dotted lines) of the points about the line; each deviation equals the difference between the observed value of y and the corresponding point on the line, $a + bx$.

In this example,

$$b = 8.96/205.38 = 0.043615$$

and:

$$a = 3.0025 - 0.043615 \times 66.875 = 0.0857$$

Thus the dependence of plasma volume on body weight is described by:

$$\text{Plasma volume} = 0.0857 + 0.0436 \times \text{weight}$$

which is shown in Figure 9.1. The regression line is drawn by calculating the coordinates of two points which lie on it. For example:

$$x=60,\ y=0.0857+0.0436\times 60=2.7$$

and

$$x=70,\ y=0.0857+0.0436\times 70=3.1$$

As a check, the line should pass through the point $(\bar{x}, \bar{y})=(66.9, 3.0)$.

The calculated values for a and b are sample estimates of the values of the intercept and slope from the regression line describing the linear association between x and y in the whole population. They are, therefore, subject to sampling variation and their precision is measured by their standard errors.

$$\text{s.e. (a)}=s\sqrt{\left[\frac{1}{n}+\frac{\bar{x}^2}{\Sigma(x-\bar{x})^2}\right]} \quad \text{and} \quad \text{s.e. (b)}=\frac{s}{\sqrt{\Sigma(x-\bar{x})^2}}$$

where

$$s=\sqrt{\left[\frac{\Sigma(y-\bar{y})^2-\text{b}^2\Sigma(x-\bar{x})^2}{(n-2)}\right]}$$

s is the **standard deviation of the points about the line**. It has $(n-2)$ degrees of freedom.

$$s=\sqrt{\frac{0.6780-0.0436^2\times 205.38}{6}}=0.2189$$

$$\text{s.e. (a)}=0.2819\sqrt{\left[\frac{1}{8}+\frac{66.9^2}{205.38}\right]}=1.3197$$

and

$$\text{s.e. (b)}=\frac{0.2189}{\sqrt{205.38}}=0.0153$$

Significance test

A t test is used to test whether b differs significantly from a specified value, denoted by β (Greek letter beta).

$$t=\frac{\text{b}-\beta}{\text{s.e. (b)}},\quad \text{d.f.}=n-2$$

In particular it may be used to test whether b is significantly different from zero. This is exactly equivalent to the t test of $r=0$. Testing this for the plasma volume and body weight example gives:

$$t=\frac{\mathrm{b}-0}{\text{s.e. (b)}}=\frac{0.0436}{0.0153}=2.85$$

which, apart from rounding error, is the same as the t value of 2.86, obtained above for the correlation coefficient. Thus plasma volume does increase significantly ($P<0.05$) with body weight.

Prediction

In some situations it may be useful to use the regression equation to predict the value of y for a particular value of x, say x'. The predicted value is:

$$y'=\mathrm{a}+\mathrm{b}x'$$

and its standard error is:

$$\text{s.e. }(y')=s\sqrt{\left[1+\frac{1}{n}+\frac{(x'-\bar{x})^2}{\Sigma(x-\bar{x})^2}\right]}$$

This standard error is least when x' is close to the mean, $\bar{x}$. In general, one should be reluctant to use the regression line for predicting values outside the range of x in the original data, as the linear relationship will not necessarily hold true beyond the range over which it has been fitted.

In the example, the measurement of plasma volume is time-consuming and so, in some circumstances, it may be convenient to predict it from the body weight. For instance, the predicted plasma volume for a man weighing 66 kg is:

$$0.0832+0.0436\times 66=2.96 \text{ litres}$$

and its standard error equals:

$$0.2189\sqrt{\left[1+\frac{1}{8}+\frac{(66-66.9)^2}{205.38}\right]}=0.23 \text{ litres.}$$

Assumptions

There are two assumptions underlying the method of linear regression. The first is that, for any value of x, y is normally distributed. The second is that the magnitude of the scatter of the points about the line is the same throughout the length of the line. This scatter is measured by the standard deviation, *s*, of the points about the line as defined above. A change of scale may be appropriate if either of these assumptions does not hold, or if the relationship seems non-linear (*see* Chapter 19). Non-linear relationships are also discussed in Chapter 10.

Use of calculators

Some calculators have an automatic correlation and linear regression facility (*see* Chapter 1), which avoids the necessity for much of the tedious calculation described above.

CHAPTER 10

Multiple Regression

Introduction

Situations frequently occur in which we are interested in the dependency of a variable on *several* explanatory variables, not just one. For example, 100 women attending an antenatal clinic took part in a study to identify variables associated with birth weight of the child, with the eventual aim of predicting women 'at risk' of having a low birth weight baby. The results showed that birth weight was significantly related to age of mother, height of mother, parity, period of gestation, and family income, but that these variables were not independent. For example, height of mother and period of gestation were positively correlated. The joint influence of the variables, taking account of possible correlations among them, may be investigated using **multiple regression**, which will be discussed in the context of this example.

To introduce the methods needed for multiple regression, an alternative formulation for simple linear regression equivalent to that described in Chapter 9, but better suited to generalization, will first be described. This will then be extended to more than one explanatory variable. Details of the calculations will not be given as the analysis would almost certainly be carried out using a computer package. The methodology is fairly complex and some readers may prefer to omit this chapter at a first reading.

Analysis of variance approach to simple linear regression

Consider the relationship of birth weight with height of mother. A scatter diagram suggested that this was linear. The correlation coefficient was 0.26 ($P<0.01$).

Linear regression gives the equation of the straight line that best describes the relationship as:

$$\text{Birth weight} = a + b \text{ height of mother}$$

where a and b are calculated so as to minimize the sum of squared deviations of the points about this line. The sum of squared deviations about the line which remains after this minimization process has been carried out is called the **residual sum of squares**. This is less than the total sum of squares of the overall variation in the birth weight by an amount which is called the sum of squares **explained by the regression** of birth weight on height of mother, or simply the **regression sum of squares**. This splitting of the total sum of squares of the overall variation in birth weight into two parts can be laid out in an analysis of variance table (Table 10.1). There is 1 degree of freedom for the regression and $n-2=98$ degrees of freedom for the residual.

Table 10.1 Analysis of variance for the linear regression of birth weight on height of mother ($n=100$).

Source of variation	Sum of squares (SS)	Degrees of freedom (d.f.)	Mean square (MS = SS/d.f.)	$F=\frac{\text{MS regression}}{\text{MS residual}}$
Regression on height of mother	1.48	1	1.4800	7.11, $P<0.01$
Residual	20.39	98	0.2081	
Total	21.87	99		

If there were no real association between the variables, then the regression mean square would be about the same size as the residual mean square, while if the variables were associated it would be larger. This is tested using an F test, as described in Chapter 8.

$$F=\frac{\text{regression mean square}}{\text{residual mean square}}, \quad \text{d.f.}=(1, n-2)$$

F should be about 1 if there is not an association, and larger if there is. This F test is equivalent to the t tests of $b=0$ and $r=0$ described in Chapter 9, the value of F equalling t^2. In this example $F=1.4800/0.2081=7.11$ with (1,98) degrees of freedom. From Table A4, the 1% point for $F(1,60)$ is 7.08 and for $F(1,120)$ is 6.85. The 1% point for $F(1,98)$ is therefore between 7.08 and 6.85 and so $F=7.11$ is significant at the 1% level.

Relationship between correlation coefficient and analysis of variance table

The analysis of variance table gives an alternative interpretation of the correlation coefficient; the square of the correlation coefficient, r^2, equals the regression sum of squares divided by the total sum of squares

($0.26^2 = 0.0676 = 1.48/21.87$) and thus is the proportion of the total variation that has been explained by the regression. We can say that height of the mother accounts for 6.76% of the total variation in birth weight.

Multiple regression with two variables

Consider now the relationship of birth weight with the two variables: height of mother and period of gestation. Scatter diagrams suggested that the relationship of birth weight with each of these was linear. The correlations were 0.26 ($P<0.01$) and 0.39 ($P<0.001$) respectively. The joint relationship can be represented by the **multiple regression equation**,

$$y = a + b_1 x_1 + b_2 x_2$$

which in this example is:

$$\text{Birth weight} = a + b_1 \text{ height of mother} + b_2 \text{ period of gestation}$$

This means that for any period of gestation, birth weight is linearly related to height of mother, and also, for any height of mother, birth weight is linearly related to period of gestation. b_1 and b_2 are called **partial regression coefficients** and the corresponding correlations are **partial correlations**. Note that b_1 and b_2 will be different to the ordinary regression coefficients unless the two explanatory variables are unrelated.

Although it is no longer easy to visualize the regression, the principles involved are the same. Each observed birth weight is compared with ($a + b_1$ height of mother $+ b_2$ gestation). a, b_1 and b_2 are chosen to minimize the sum of squares of these differences or, in other words, the variation about the regression. The results are laid out in an analysis of variance table (Table 10.2). There are now 2 degrees of freedom for the regression as there are two explanatory variables.

Table 10.2 Analysis of variance for the multiple regression of birth weight on height of mother and period of gestation.

Source of variation	SS	d.f.	MS	$F = \frac{\text{MS regression}}{\text{MS residual}}$
Regression on height of mother *and* period of gestation	4.43	2	2.2150	12.32, $P<0.001$
Residual	17.44	97	0.1798	
Total	21.87	99		

The F test for this regression is 12.32 with (2,97) degrees of freedom and is significant at the 0.1% level. The regression accounts for 20.26% (4.43/21.87) of the total variation. This proportion equals R^2, where $R=\sqrt{0.2026}=0.45$ is defined as the **multiple correlation coefficient**. R is always positive as no direction can be attached to a correlation based on more than one variable.

The sum of squares due to the regression of birth weight on both height of mother and period of gestation comprises the sum of squares explained by height of mother (as calculated in the simple linear regression) plus the *extra* sum of squares explained by the period of gestation after allowing for height of mother (Table 10.3a). This extra variation can also be tested for significance using an F test. The residual mean square from the multiple regression is used.

$$F=2.95/0.1798=16.41,\ \text{d.f.}=(1,97),\ P<0.001$$

Thus the model with both variables is an improvement over the model with just height of mother, because the effect of period of gestation is significant even when height of mother is taken into account.

Table 10.3 Individual contributions of height of mother and period of gestation to the multiple regression including both variables.

(a) Height of mother entered into multiple regression first.

Source of variation	SS	d.f.	MS	$F=\frac{\text{MS regression}}{\text{MS residual}}$
Height of mother	1.48	1	1.48	8.23, $P<0.01$
Gestation adjusting for height	2.95	1	2.95	16.41, $P<0.001$
Height of mother and period of gestation	4.43	2		

(b) Period of gestation entered into multiple regression first.

Source of variation	SS	d.f.	MS	$F=\frac{\text{MS regression}}{\text{MS residual}}$
Period of gestation	3.33	1	3.33	18.52, $P<0.001$
Height adjusting for gestation	1.10	1	1.10	6.12, $P<0.025$
Height of mother and period of gestation	4.43	2		

Alternatively, the sum of squares explained by the regression with both variables comprises the sum of squares explained by period of gestation (calculated by simple linear regression) plus the extra sum of squares due to height of mother after allowing for period of gestation. This is shown in Table 10.3(b). Again, we see that the model with both variables is an improvement over the model with just period of gestation, since the effect of height of mother is significant even when period of gestation is taken into account.

The two orders of breaking down the combined regression sum of squares from Table 10.2 into the separate sums of squares do not give the same component sums of squares (Tables 10.3a and b) because the explanatory variables (height of mother and period of gestation) are themselves correlated.

Multiple regression with several variables

Multiple regression can be extended to any number of variables, although it is recommended that the number be kept reasonably small, as with larger numbers the interpretation becomes increasingly more complex. Some variables, such as age and sex, may be essential for inclusion in the multiple regression equation because it is considered necessary to adjust for their effects before investigating other relationships. The inclusion of other variables may be based on the strengths of their associations with the dependent variable. The object should be to achieve a balance between, on the one hand, including sufficient variables to obtain the best possible agreement between the multiple regression equation and the data and, on the other hand, not including so many variables as to make the relationship too complex to interpret. The selection of variables can be made in one of three ways.

1 Step-up regression. Simple linear regressions are carried out on each of the explanatory variables. The one accounting for the largest percentage of variation is chosen and kept as the first variable. Multiple regressions with two variables are then carried out adding each of the other explanatory variables in turn. The two-variable regression accounting for the largest percentage of variation is chosen. The process continues, an additional variable being selected at each stage. It stops when either the extra variation accounted for by adding a further variable is non-significant for all the remaining variables *or* when a preset limit for the maximum number of variables in the multiple regression has been reached.

2 Step-down regression. A multiple regression is performed using all the explanatory variables. Variables are then dropped, one at a time. At each stage, the variable chosen for exclusion is that which makes the least contribution to the explained variation. The process continues until all remaining variables are significant, *or*, if the number of remaining variables is still too many, until a preset limit for the maximum number of variables in the equation has been reached.

3 Optimal combination regression. The stepwise regressions of methods 1 and 2 do not necessarily reach the same final choice, even if they end up with the same number of explanatory variables incl ded. Neither of them will necessarily choose the best possible regression for a given number of explanatory variables. A preferable procedure is to find which single variable is best, then which pair of variables is best, then which trio, etc., by performing regressions of all possible combinations. Note that, for example, the best pair will not necessarily include the best single variable, although often it does.

Multiple regression with discrete explanatory variables

It is often desirable to include discrete as well as continuous explanatory variables in a multiple regression analysis. For example, in the birth weight study, six of the 100 women had a mycoplasma infection during pregnancy, and on average the birth weight of their babies was lower. This factor is included by defining a **dummy variable** for infection which equals 1 for women who had a mycoplasma infection and zero for women who did not. The regression equation is:

$$\text{Birth weight} = a + b_1 \text{ height of mother} + b_2 \text{ period of gestation} + b_3 \text{ infection}$$

This is equivalent to a pair of equations:

(a) Birth weight $= a + b_1$ height of mother $+ b_2$ period of gestation $+ b_3$ for women who had a mycoplasma infection, and

(b) Birth weight $= a + b_1$ height of mother $+ b_2$ period of gestation for women who did not have an infection

The coefficient b_3 measures the average difference in birth weight of babies born to mothers who had a mycoplasma infection compared to mothers of the same height and with the same period of gestation who did not have the infection. The additional sum of squares due to mycoplasma infection is found by exactly the same methods as described above. It is the difference between the sum of squares due to the three-variables multiple regression including the dummy variable representing infection, and that due to the regression on just height of mother and period of gestation. It has 1 degree of freedom and is tested for significance using an F test.

Mycoplasma infection is a factor with two levels, presence or absence. Factors with more than two levels, such as age-group, are included by the introduction of a series of dummy variables to describe the differences. If a factor has k levels, $k-1$ dummy variables are needed and the associated degrees of freedom equal $k-1$. For details see Armitage & Berry (1987).

Multiple regression with non-linear explanatory variables

It is often found that the relationship between the dependent variable and an explanatory variable is non-linear. There are three possible ways of incorporating such an explanatory variable in the multiple regression equation. The first and most versatile method is to redefine the variable into distinct subgroups and include it as a factor with a level corresponding to each subgroup, as described in the section above, rather than as a continuous variable. For example, age could be subdivided into five-year age-groups. The relationship with age would then be based on a comparison of the means of the dependent variable in each age-group and would make no assumption about the exact form of the relationship with age. At the initial stages of an analysis, it is often useful to include an explanatory variable in both forms, as a continuous variable and as a factor. The difference between the two associated sums of squares can then be used to assess whether there is an important non-linear component to the relationship. For most purposes, a subdivision into 3–5 groups, depending on the sample size, is adequate to investigate non-linearity of the relationship.

A second possibility is to find a suitable transformation for the explanatory variable. For example, in the birth weight study, it was found that birth weight was linearly related to the logarithm of family income rather than to family income itself. The use of transformations is discussed more fully in Chapter 19. The third possibility is to find an algebraic description of the relationship. For example, it may be quadratic, in which case both the variable (x) and its square (x^2) would be added into the equation.

Relationship between multiple regression and analysis of variance

There is a large overlap between multiple regression and analysis of variance. A multiple regression where all of the explanatory variables are discrete is, in fact, the same as an analysis of variance with several factors. The two approaches give identical results. In such a situation it is recommended that the choice of method be based on the computer programs available and their relative ease of use.

Another closely related technique, which will not be described here in detail, is **analysis of covariance** (Armitage & Berry 1987). It is an alternative but equivalent approach to investigating differences between groups when there are also continuous explanatory variables. An example is the problem described above of comparing birth weights of babies between mothers who had a mycoplasma infection during pregnancy and those who did not. Height of mother and period of gestation were additional explanatory variables and would be called **covariates** in this context. Note that analysis of covariance is sometimes included as part of the analysis of variance procedure in computer packages.

Multivariate analysis

Multiple regression, analysis of variance, logistic regression (*see* Chapter 13) and log linear models (*see* Chapter 13) are often referred to as *multivariate* methods, since they investigate how a dependent variable is related to more than one explanatory variable. In the strict statistical sense, however, **multivariate analysis** means the study of how several *dependent* variables vary together. The four methods most appropriate to medical research will briefly be described. For more detail see Armitage and Berry (1987).

Principal component analysis is a method used to find a few combinations of variables, called components, that adequately explain the overall observed variation, and thus to reduce the complexity of the data. **Discriminant analysis** is a method used to find a single combination of variables, called the **discriminant function**, that best distinguishes between different subgroups. This function is then used to predict to which subgroup a new individual is likely to belong. For example, it has been used to predict infants at risk of cot death. **Factor analysis** is a method commonly used in the analysis of psychological tests. It seeks to explain how the responses to the various test items may be influenced by a number of underlying *factors*, such as emotion, rational thinking, etc. Finally, **cluster analysis** is a method which examines a collection of variables to see if individuals can be formed into any natural system of groups. Techniques used include those of **numerical taxonomy**, principal components and **correspondance analysis**.

CHAPTER 11

Probability

Introduction

Probability has already been used several times in the preceding chapters, its meaning being clear from the context. It is now time to introduce it more formally and to give the rules for manipulating it. Although probability is a concept used in everyday life, and one with which we have an intuitive familiarity, it is difficult to define exactly. The **frequentist definition** is usually used in statistics. This states that the **probability** of the occurrence of a particular event equals the proportion of times that the event would (or does) occur in a large number of similar repeated trials. It has a value between 0 and 1, equalling 0 if the event can never occur and 1 if it is certain to occur. A probability may also be expressed as a percentage, taking a value between 0% and 100%. For example, suppose a coin is tossed thousands of times and in half the tosses it lands head up and in half it lands tail up. The probability of getting a head at any one toss would be defined as one-half, or 50%.

An alternative is the **subjective definition**, where the size of the probability simply represents one's degree of belief in the occurrence of an event, or in an hypothesis. This definition corresponds more closely with everyday usage and is the foundation of the **Bayesian** approach to statistics. In this approach, the investigator assigns a **prior probability** to the event (or hypothesis) under investigation. The study is then carried out, the data collected and the probability modified in the light of the results obtained. The revised probability is called the **posterior probability**. The statistical methods arising from this approach are quite different, and not widely used. For more details see Lindley (1965).

Probability calculations

There are just two rules underlying the calculation of all probabilities. These are:

1 The **multiplicative rule** for the probability of the occurrence of *both* of two events, A and B, and;

2 The **additive rule** for the occurrence of *either* event A *or* event B (*or both*).

Multiplicative rule

Consider a couple who plan to have two children. There are four possible combinations for the sexes of these children, as shown in Table 11.1. Each combination is equally likely and so has a probability of 1/4.

Table 11.1 The possible combinations for the sexes of two children, with their probabilities

	Second child	
	Boy 1/2	Girl 1/2
First child		
Boy 1/2	1/4 (boy, boy)	1/4 (boy, girl)
Girl 1/2	1/4 (girl, boy)	1/4 (girl, girl)

In fact each of these probabilities of 1/4 derives from the individual probabilities of the sexes of each of the children. Consider in more detail the probability that both children are girls. The probability that the first child is a girl is 1/2. There is then a probability of 1/2 of this (i.e. $1/2$ of $1/2 = 1/4$) that the second child will *also* be a girl. Thus:

$$\begin{aligned}\text{Prob (both children are girls)} &= \text{prob (first child is a girl)} \\ &\quad \times \text{prob (second child is a girl)} \\ &= 1/2 \times 1/2 = 1/4\end{aligned}$$

The general rule for the probability of both of two events is:

Prob (A *and* B) = prob (A) × prob (B given that A has occurred)

Prob (B given that A has occurred) is called a **conditional probability**, as it is the probability of the occurrence of event B conditional upon the occurrence of event A. If the likelihood of event B is unaffected by the occurrence or non-occurrence of event A, and vice versa, events A and B are said to be **independent** and the rule simplifies to:

Prob (A *and* B) = Prob (A) × prob (B), if A and B are independent

The sexes of children are independent events as the probability that the next child is a girl is uninfluenced by the sexes of the previous children. An example with dependent events is the probability that a young girl in India is both anaemic and malnourished, since she is much more likely to be anaemic if she is malnourished than if she is not.

Additive rule

Prob (A *or* B *or* both) = prob (A) + prob (B) − prob (both)

This is explained in the context of a particular example. Consider an area in South America where the probability of having hookworm infestation is 0.5 and the probability of having schistosomiasis is 0.6. Clearly the probability of having either hookworm or schistosomiasis or both is not the sum, $0.5 + 0.6 = 1.1$, since probabilities cannot be larger than one. The problem is that the probability of having both hookworm and schistosomiasis has been counted twice, once as part of the probability of having hookworm and once as part of the probability of having schistosomiasis. The correct calculation is:

prob (hookworm or schistosomiasis or both) =
prob (hookworm) + prob (schistosomiasis) − prob (both)

If the two diseases occur independently of each other:

$$\text{prob (both)} = 0.5 \times 0.6 = 0.3$$

and

$$\text{prob (hookworm or schistosomiasis or both)} = 0.5 + 0.6 - 0.3 = 0.8.$$

CHAPTER 12

Proportions

Introduction

The methods described in Chapters 4–10 are for continuous variables. We now consider methods appropriate for proportions, which are discrete variables. We begin by describing the sampling distribution of a proportion which is based on the so-called binomial distribution, and we describe later how this binomial distribution can often be approximated by the familiar normal distribution.

Binomial distribution

A proportion is made up from a **binary variable**, where for each individual in the sample the value is one of two alternatives which we can label A and B. For example, a patient survives (A) or dies (B), a specimen is positive (A) or negative (B), or a child has (A) or has not (B) been vaccinated. The **proportion** (p) of A's is the number (r) of A's divided by the total number in the sample.

$$p = r/n$$

The number (and proportion) of A's observed in the sample is, of course, subject to sampling variation (*see* Chapter 3), different samples being likely to give different values. The sampling distribution is called the **binomial distribution** and this can be calculated from the sample size, n, and the *population* proportion, π, as shown in Example 12.1. π (Greek letter pi; not related here to the mathematical constant 3.1459) is the probability that the response for any one individual is A.

Example 12.1
A man and woman each with sickle cell trait (AS; that is, heterozygous for the sickle cell [S] and normal [A] haemoglobin genes) have four children. What is the probability that none, one, two, three, or four of the children have sickle cell disease (SS)?

For each child the probability of being SS is the probability of having inherited the S gene from each parent, which is $0.5 \times 0.5 = 0.25$ by the multiplicative rule of probabilities (Chapter 11). The probability of not being SS (i.e. of being AS or AA) is therefore 0.75. We shall call being SS alternative A and not being SS alternative B, so $\pi = 0.25$.

The probability that none of the children is SS (i.e. $r = 0$) is $0.75 \times 0.75 \times 0.75 \times 0.75 = 0.75^4 = 0.3164$, where 0.75^4 means 0.75 multiplied together four times. This is by the multiplicative rule of probabilities.

The probability that exactly one child is SS is the probability that (first child SS; second, third, fourth not SS) or (second child SS; first, third, fourth not SS) or (third child SS; first, second, fourth not SS) or (fourth child SS; first, second, third not SS). Each of these four possibilities has probability 0.25×0.75^3 (multiplicative rule) and since they cannot occur together the probability of one or other of them occurring is $4 \times 0.25 \times 0.75^3 = 0.4219$, by the additive rule of probabilities.

In similar fashion, one can calculate the probability that exactly two, three, or four children are SS by working out in each case the different possible arrangements within the family and adding together their probabilities. This gives the probabilities shown in Table 12.1. Note that the sum of these probabilities is 1, which it has to be as one of the alternatives must occur. The probabilities are also illustrated as a probability distribution in Figure 12.1. This is the binomial probability distribution for $\pi = 0.25$ and $n = 4$.

Table 12.1 Calculation of the probabilities of the possible numbers of children who have inherited sickle cell (SS) disease, in a family of four children where both parents have the sickle cell trait. (The probability that an individual child inherits sickle cell disease is 0.25.)

No. of children		No. of ways in which combination could occur	Probability
With SS	Without SS		
0	4	1	$1 \times 1 \times 0.75^4 = 0.3164$
1	3	4	$4 \times 0.25 \times 0.75^3 = 0.4219$
2	2	6	$6 \times 0.25^2 \times 0.75^2 = 0.2109$
3	1	4	$4 \times 0.25^3 \times 0.75 = 0.0469$
4	0	1	$1 \times 0.25^4 \times 1 = 0.0039$
			Total = 1.0000

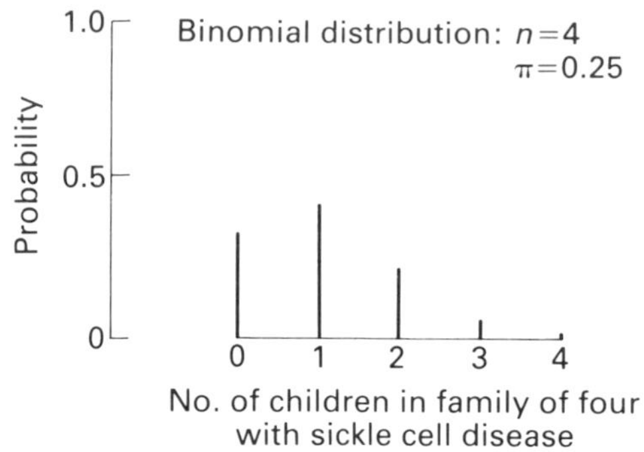

Figure 12.1 Probability distribution of the number of children in a family of four with sickle cell disease where both parents have the sickle cell trait. The probability that a child inherits sickle cell disease is 0.25.

General formula for binomial probabilities

The general formula for the probability of getting exactly r A's in a sample of n individuals when the probability of A for each individual is π is:

$$\text{Prob}\ (r\text{ A's}) = \frac{n!}{r!(n-r)!}\pi^r(1-\pi)^{n-r}$$

The first part of the formula represents the number of possible ways in which r A's could be observed in a sample of size n, and the second part equals the probability of each of these ways. The exclamation mark denotes the *factorial* of the number and means all the integers from the number down to 1 multiplied together. (0! is defined to equal 1.) π^r means π multiplied together r times or, in mathematical terminology, π to the power r. Any number to the power zero is defined to equal 1. For example, applying the formula in the above example to calculate the probability that exactly two out of the four children are SS gives:

$$\text{prob}\ (2\text{ SS's}) = \frac{4!}{2!(4-2)!}0.25^2(1-0.25)^{(4-2)}$$

$$= \frac{4 \times 3 \times 2 \times 1}{2 \times 1 \times 2 \times 1} \times 0.25^2 \times 0.75^2$$

$$= 6 \times 0.25^2 \times 0.75^2 = 0.2109$$

Many calculators have keys for factorial and for the power of a number. If not, the first part of the formula may be more easily calculated using the following expression, where $(n-r)!$ has been cancelled into $n!$

$$\frac{n!}{r!(n-r)!}=\frac{n\times(n-1)\times(n-2)\times\ \ldots\ \times(n-r+1)}{r\times(r-1)\times\ \ldots\ \times 3\times 2\times 1}$$

For example, if $n=18$ and $r=5$, $(n-r+1)=18-5+1=14$ and the expression equals:

$$\frac{18\times 17\times 16\times 15\times 14}{5\times 4\times 3\times 2\times 1}=\frac{1028160}{120}=8568$$

The interested reader may like to practise the application of the above formula by checking the calculations presented in Tables 12.1 and 12.3. Note that when π equals 0.5, $(1-\pi)$ also equals 0.5 and the second part of the formula simplifies to 0.5^n.

Properties of the binomial distribution

Figure 12.2 shows examples of the binomial distribution for various values of π and n. These distributions have been illustrated for r, the number of A's in the sample, although they apply equally to p, the proportion of A's. For example, when the sample size, n, equals 5, the possible values for r are 0, 1, 2, 3, 4 or 5, and the horizontal axis has been labelled accordingly. The corresponding proportions are 0, 0.2, 0.4, 0.6, 0.8 and 1 respectively. Relabelling the horizontal axis with these values would give the binomial distribution for p. Note that, although p is a fraction, its sampling distribution is discrete and not continuous, since it may take only a limited number of values for any given sample size.

Since the binomial distribution is the *sampling* distribution for the number (or proportion) of A's, its mean equals the population mean and its standard deviation represents the standard error, which measures how closely the sample value estimates the population value. The population means and standard errors are given in Table 12.2 for the number, proportion and

Table 12.2 Population mean and standard error for the number, proportion, and percentage of A's in a sample.

	Observed value	Population mean	Standard error
Number of A's	r	$n\pi$	$\sqrt{\{n\pi(1-\pi)\}}$
Proportion of A's	$p=r/n$	π	$\sqrt{\{\pi(1-\pi)/n\}}$
Percentage of A's	$100p$	100π	$100\sqrt{\{\pi(1-\pi)/n\}}$

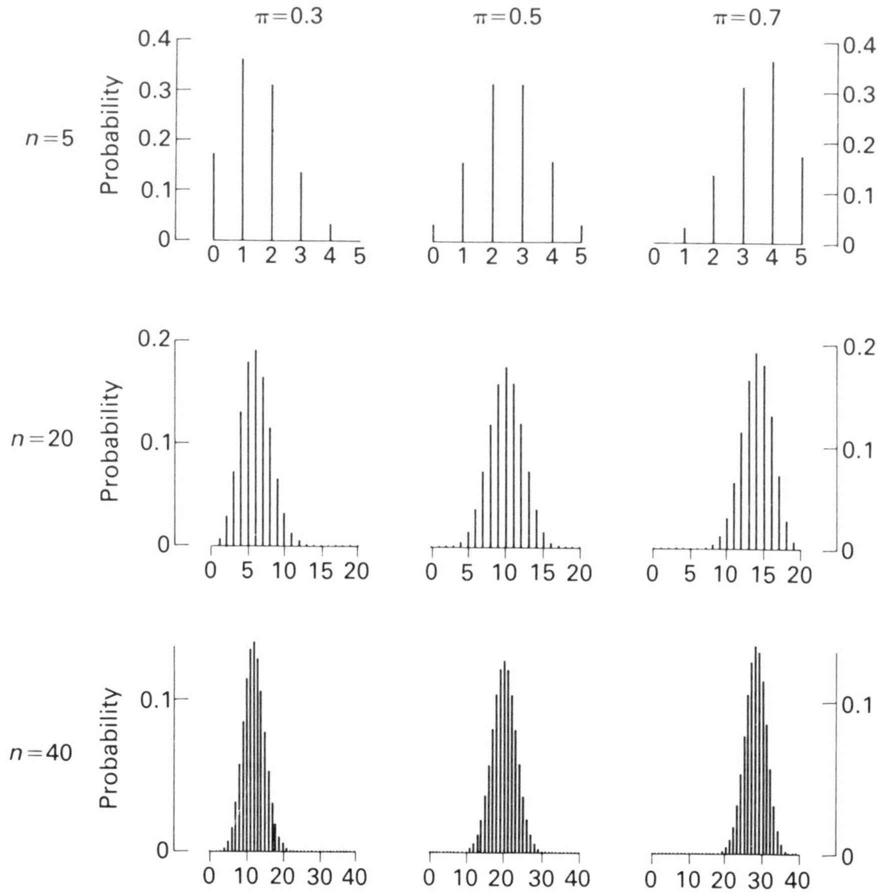

Figure 12.2 Binomial distribution for various values of π and n. The horizontal scale in each diagram shows values of r.

percentage of A's. The percentage is, of course, just the proportion multiplied by 100.

Significance test for a single proportion using binomial distribution

Consider the results of a clinical trial to compare two analgesics, A and B. Twelve migraine sufferers were given drug A on one occasion and drug B on another, the order in which the drugs were given being chosen at random for each patient. The patients were each asked which drug gave them greater relief. Nine patients responded drug A, and three responded drug B. Does this mean that on average drug A is really more effective, or could the difference have been due to chance?

As in Chapter 6 a significance test is used to decide which explanation is more likely. The null hypothesis is that the drugs are equally effective. If this were the case, a patient should be equally likely to respond A or B (assuming that some preference must be given). The sampling distribution for the number of A responses is therefore a binomial distribution with $\pi = 0.5$ and $n = 12$.

Recall from Chapter 6 that the significance level is the probability of getting a result as extreme as or more extreme than the result which was observed. In this example, this is the probability of nine, ten, eleven, or twelve A responses *plus* the probability of three, two, one, or zero A responses. As before, for a *two-sided* significance test we have to take both extremes of the sampling distribution into account. The binomial distribution is symmetrical for $\pi = 0.5$. Thus, for example, the probability of getting three A responses is the same as the probability of getting nine A responses, just as in 12 tosses of a coin one is as likely to get three heads and nine tails as to get nine heads and three tails.

The probabilities of nine, ten, eleven, or twelve A responses are given in Table 12.3 and total 0.0729. The probability of extreme responses (3, 2, 1, 0) in the other direction is also 0.0729. Therefore the probability of getting a result as extreme as or more extreme than nine A responses from 12 patients, by chance, is 0.1458 or 14.58%. Since this probability is quite large we conclude that the trial has not demonstrated a significant difference in effectiveness between the drugs.

Calculation of significance level when $\pi \neq 0.5$

In general, we can use the same method to test the significance of the difference of any sample proportion, p, from any null hypothesis value, π, for

Table 12.3 Calculation of significance level for a clinical trial in which nine out of 12 patients preferred drug A to drug B.

Number of preferences for drug A		Probability
Observed result:	9	$220 \times 0.5^{12} = 0.0537$
More extreme results:	10	$66 \times 0.5^{12} = 0.0161$
	11	$12 \times 0.5^{12} = 0.0029$
	12	$0.5^{12} = 0.0002$
Total: 9, 10, 11, 12		0.0729
Other tail: 3, 2, 1, 0		0.0729
Total (two-sided significance level)		0.1458

the proportion in the population. When π is not 0.5 the binomial distribution is asymmetrical, however, and the probabilities in the upper and lower tails are not the same. One can then calculate the significance level by adding together (i) the probabilities of the observed sample value and of the more extreme values in the same direction, and (ii) the probabilities of each value in the opposite direction for which the probability is less than that for the observed sample value. Alternatively, one can simply take the sum of probabilities in the observed direction, i.e. probability (i), and double it. The results will be different, but the choice is unlikely, in practice, to affect the assessment of whether the observed difference is due to chance or to a real effect. Neither method is clearly superior to the other, but the second method is simpler to carry out.

Normal approximation to binomial distribution

When the sample size, n, is large it can be tedious to calculate probabilities for each value in the tails of the binomial distribution in order to perform a significance test as above. Fortunately, as n increases the binomial distribution becomes very close to a normal distribution (*see* Figure 12.2). In fact the normal distribution is a reasonable approximation to the binomial distribution if both $n\pi$ and $n - n\pi$ are 5 or more. The approximating normal distribution has the same mean and standard deviation as the binomial distribution (*see* Table 12.2).

Significance tests and confidence intervals using normal approximation

The normal distribution can be used for significance tests of proportions in exactly the same way as it was used for significance tests of means (*see* Chapters 6 and 7), and it can also be used to construct confidence intervals.

Significance test for a single proportion

The normal test for a single proportion uses the formula:

$$z = \frac{p - \pi}{\text{s.e.}(p)} = \frac{p - \pi}{\sqrt{\{\pi(1-\pi)/n\}}}$$

For example, in the clinical trial to compare two analgesics described above, the proportion of patients preferring drug A was $9/12 = 0.75$ compared to the null hypothesis value $\pi = 0.5$.

$$z = \frac{0.75 - 0.5}{\sqrt{\{0.5 \times 0.5/12\}}} = 1.73$$

The value 1.73 lies between the 5% and 10% percentage points of the standard normal distribution (Table A2). Its exact significance level can be found from Table A1 and is $2 \times 0.0418 = 0.0836$ or 8.36%. This is appreciably smaller than the corresponding value of 14.58% calculated using the binomial probabilities. The reason for this is that we have used a continuous distribution, the normal distribution, to approximate the binomial distribution, which is discrete. This situation is corrected by the introduction of what is called a **continuity correction** into the formula for the normal test.

The normal test with continuity correction is:

$$z = \frac{|p - \pi| - 1/(2n)}{\sqrt{\{\pi(1-\pi)/n\}}}$$

where $|p - \pi|$ means the absolute value of $p - \pi$ or, in other words, the value of $p - \pi$ ignoring the minus sign if it is negative.

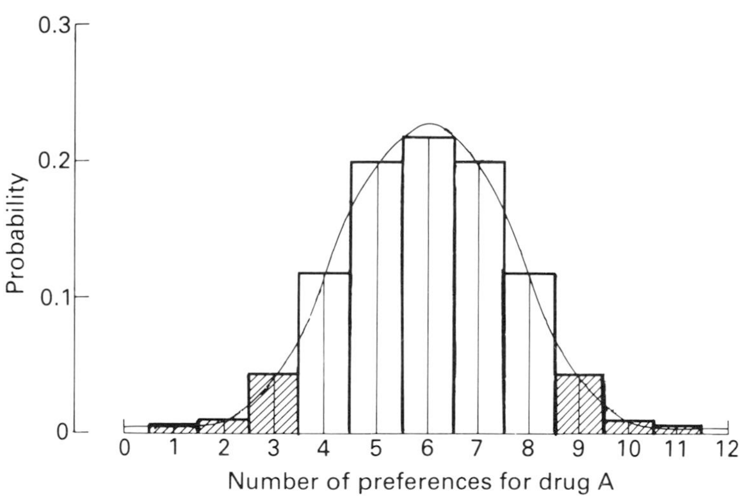

Figure 12.3 Binomial distribution ($n = 12$, $\pi = 0.5$) for the number of patients preferring drug A, together with the approximating normal distribution. The shaded area shows the probability of observing a number of preferences for A as extreme as or more extreme than nine and illustrates the use of the continuity correction.

The effect of the continuity correction is to reduce the value of z and to improve the agreement with the binomial test. In the example, the z value with continuity correction is:

$$z = \frac{|0.75 - 0.5| - 1/24}{\sqrt{\{0.5 \times 0.5/12\}}} = 1.44$$

From Table A1 the significance level for $z = 1.44$ is $2 \times 0.0749 = 0.1498$ or 14.98% which agrees much better with the value of 14.58% from the binomial test.

The rationale of the continuity correction can be understood quite well from Figure 12.3, where the normal and binomial distributions are superimposed. What we are doing when we use the continuity correction is effectively to calculate the areas for the normal distribution below $r = 3.5$ and above $r = 8.5$, instead of below $r = 3$ and above $r = 9$. It can be seen that this gives better agreement with the shaded areas representing the tail probabilities of the binomial distribution.

Confidence interval for a single proportion

Using the binomial distribution to derive a confidence interval for a proportion is complicated. Intervals are, however, tabulated in the *Geigy Scientific Tables* (1982) for various proportions and for samples up to size 100. An alternative approach is to obtain an approximate formula using the normal distribution and methods similar to those described in Chapter 5. This gives:

$$\text{c.i.} = p \pm z' \times \text{s.e.}, \quad \text{s.e.} = \sqrt{\{p(1-p)/n\}}$$

where z' is the appropriate percentage point of the standard normal distribution. For example, for a 95% confidence interval $z' = 1.96$. This formula does not have a continuity correction and is suitable only when both np and $n - np$ are 10 or more.

Significance test for comparing two proportions

The normal test to compare two sample proportions, $p_1 = r_1/n_1$ and $p_2 = r_2/n_2$ is based on:

$$z = \frac{p_1 - p_2}{\text{s.e.}(p_1 - p_2)}$$

where the standard error of $p_1 - p_2$, under the null hypothesis that the population proportions are equal (i.e. $\pi_1 = \pi_2 = \pi$), is:

$$\text{s.e.}(p_1 - p_2) = \sqrt{\{\pi(1-\pi)(1/n_1 + 1/n_2)\}}$$

π is estimated by the *overall* proportion in both samples, that is by:

$$p = \frac{r_1 + r_2}{n_1 + n_2}$$

As in the case of a single proportion the test is improved by inclusion of a **continuity correction**. The formula is then:

$$z = \frac{|p_1 - p_2| - \{1/(2n_1) + 1/(2n_2)\}}{\sqrt{\{p(1-p)(1/n_1 + 1/n_2)\}}}, \quad p = \frac{r_1 + r_2}{n_1 + n_2}$$

(As before, $|p_1 - p_2|$ means the *size* of the difference ignoring its sign.) This normal test is a valid approximation provided that *either* $n_1 + n_2$ is greater than 40 *or* n_1p, $n_1 - n_1p$, n_2p and $n_2 - n_2p$ are all 5 or more. The exact test described in Chapter 14 should be used when this condition is not satisfied.

Confidence interval for difference between two proportions

An approximate confidence interval for the difference between two proportions is:

$$\text{c.i.} = (p_1 - p_2) \pm (z' \times \text{s.e.}), \quad \text{s.e.} = \sqrt{\{p_1(1-p_1)/n_1 + p_2(1-p_2)/n_2\}}$$

where z' is the appropriate percentage point of the normal distribution. This approximation is likely to be reasonable if n_1p_1, $n_1 - n_1p_1$, n_2p_2 and $n_2 - n_2p_2$ are each greater than 10 and will improve as these numbers get larger.

Example 12.2

Consider the following results from an influenza vaccination trial carried out during an epidemic. Twenty out of 240 ($p_1 = 0.083$ or 8.3%) persons given real vaccine contracted influenza compared to 80 out of 220 ($p_2 = 0.364$ or 36.4%) given a placebo. Is this convincing evidence that the vaccine was effective?

The overall proportion that contracted influenza was:

$$p = \frac{20 + 80}{240 + 220} = \frac{100}{460} = 0.217 \text{ or } 21.7\%$$

and so

$$z = \frac{|0.083 - 0.364| - (1/480 + 1/440)}{\sqrt{\{0.217(1 - 0.217)(1/240 + 1/220)\}}}$$

$$= \frac{0.281 - 0.0044}{0.0385} = 7.18$$

The value 7.18 is larger than 3.29, the 0.1% percentage point for the standard normal distribution. We therefore conclude that there was a highly significant ($P < 0.001$) reduction in the risk of contracting influenza following vaccination with the real vaccine. The approximate 95% confidence interval for this reduction is:

$$(p_1 - p_2) \pm 1.96\sqrt{\{p_1(1 - p_1)/n_1 + p_2(1 - p_2)/n_2\}}$$

$$= -0.281 \pm (1.96 \times 0.037) = -0.354, \ -0.208$$

That is, the probability of contracting influenza is estimated to be lower by between 20.8% and 35.4% after receiving influenza vaccine compared to receiving the placebo.

This example is discussed again at the start of the next chapter and in the section on vaccine trials in Chapter 25, where the concept of vaccine efficacy is introduced.

CHAPTER 13

The Chi-squared Test for Contingency Tables

Introduction

The presentation of data for a single qualitative variable was described in Chapter 2. When there are two qualitative variables, the data are arranged in a **contingency table**. The categories for one variable define the rows, and the categories for the other variable define the columns. Individuals are assigned to the appropriate cell of the contingency table according to their values for the two variables. A contingency table is also used for discrete quantitative variables or for continuous quantitative variables whose values have been grouped.

A **chi-squared (χ^2) test** is used to test whether there is an association between the row variable and the column variable or, in other words, whether the distribution of individuals among the categories of one variable is independent of their distribution among the categories of the other. When the table has only two rows or two columns this is equivalent to the comparison of proportions.

2 × 2 table (comparison of two proportions)

The results of the influenza vaccination trial described in Example 12.2 are arranged in tabular form in Table 13.1(a). Of 460 adults who took part, 240 received influenza vaccination and 220 placebo vaccination. Overall 100 people contracted influenza, of whom 20 were in the vaccine group and 80 in the placebo group. Such a table of data is called a **2 × 2 contingency table**, since the two variables, namely type of vaccine and presence of influenza, both have two possible values. It is sometimes called a **fourfold table** since each subject falls into one of four possible categories.

The first step in interpreting contingency table data is to calculate appropriate proportions or percentages. Thus the percentages contracting influenza were 8.3% in the vaccine group, 36.4% in the placebo group, and 21.7% overall. We now need to decide whether this is sufficient evidence that the vaccine was effective or whether the difference could have arisen by chance.

This is done using the **chi-squared test**, which compares the observed numbers in each of the four categories in the contingency table with the numbers to be expected if there were no difference in effectiveness between the

Table 13.1 Results from an influenza vaccine trial.

(a) Observed numbers.

Influenza	Vaccine	Placebo	Total
Yes	20 (8.3%)	80 (36.4%)	100 (21.7%)
No	220	140	360
Total	240	220	460

(b) Expected numbers.

Influenza	Vaccine	Placebo	Total
Yes	52.2	47.8	100
No	187.8	172.2	360
Total	240	220	460

vaccine and placebo. Overall 100/460 people contracted influenza and, if the vaccine and the placebo were equally effective, one would expect this same proportion in each of the two groups; that is $100/460 \times 240 = 52.2$ in the vaccine group and $100/460 \times 220 = 47.8$ in the placebo group would have contracted influenza. Similarly $360/460 \times 240 = 187.8$ and $360/460 \times 220 = 172.2$ would have escaped influenza. These expected numbers are shown in Table 13.1(b). They add up to the same row and column totals as the observed numbers. The chi-squared value is obtained by calculating (observed—expected)^2/expected for each of the four cells in the contingency table and then summing them.

$$\chi^2 = \Sigma \frac{(O-E)^2}{E}, \quad \text{d.f.} = 1 \text{ for a } 2 \times 2 \text{ table}$$

The greater the differences between the observed and expected numbers, the larger the value of χ^2 and the less likely it is that the difference is due to chance. The percentage points of the chi-squared distribution are given in Table A5. The values depend on the degrees of freedom, which equal 1 for a 2×2 table.

In this example:

$$\chi^2 = \frac{(20-52.2)^2}{52.2} + \frac{(80-47.8)^2}{47.8} + \frac{(220-187.8)^2}{187.8} + \frac{(140-172.2)^2}{172.2}$$

$$= 19.86 + 21.69 + 5.52 + 6.02 = 53.09$$

53.09 is greater than 10.83, the 0.1% point for the chi-squared distribution with 1 degree of freedom. Thus the probability is less than 0.1% that such a large observed difference in the percentage contracting influenza could have arisen by chance, if there were no real difference between the vaccine and the placebo. It is therefore concluded that the vaccine is effective.

Continuity correction

Like the normal test, the chi-squared test for a 2×2 table can be improved by using a continuity correction, often called **Yates' continuity correction**. The formula becomes:

$$\chi^2 = \Sigma \frac{(|O-E|-\frac{1}{2})^2}{E}, \quad \text{d.f.} = 1$$

resulting in a smaller value for χ^2. $|O-E|$ means the absolute value of $O-E$ or, in other words, the value of $O-E$ ignoring its sign.

In the example the value for χ^2 becomes:

$$\chi^2 = \frac{(32.2-\frac{1}{2})^2}{52.2} + \frac{(32.2-\frac{1}{2})^2}{47.8} + \frac{(32.2-\frac{1}{2})^2}{187.8} + \frac{(32.2-\frac{1}{2})^2}{172.2}$$

$$= 19.25 + 21.02 + 5.35 + 5.84 = 51.46, \quad P < 0.001$$

Comparison with normal test

The normal test for comparing two proportions and the chi-squared test for a 2×2 contingency table are in fact mathematically equivalent and $\chi^2 = z^2$. This is true whether or not a continuity correction is used, provided it is used or not used in both tests. For example, from Example 12.2, z^2 (with continuity correction) $= 7.18^2 = 51.55$, which apart from rounding error is the same as the χ^2 value of 51.46 calculated above. The normal test has the advantage that confidence intervals are more readily calculated. The chi-squared test is simpler to apply, however, and it can also be extended to the comparison of several proportions and to larger contingency tables.

Note that the percentage points given in Table A5 for a chi-squared distribution with 1 degree of freedom correspond to the *two*-sided percentage points presented in Table A2 for the standard normal distribution. (The concepts of one- and two-sided tests do not extend to chi-squared tests with larger degrees of freedom as these contain multiple comparisons.)

Validity

The use of the continuity correction is always advisable although it has most effect when the expected numbers are small. When they are very small the chi-squared test (and also the normal test) is not a good enough approximation, even with a continuity correction, and the alternative **exact test** for a 2×2 table should be used (*see* Chapter 14). Cochran (1954) recommends the use of the exact test when the overall total of the table is less than 20, or when it is between 20 and 40 and the smallest of the four *expected* values is less than 5. Thus the chi-squared test is valid when the overall total is more than 40, regardless of the expected values, and when the overall total is between 20 and 40 provided all the expected values are at least 5.

Table 13.2 Generalized notation for a 2×2 contingency table.

Influenza	Vaccine	Placebo	Total
Yes	a	b	e
No	c	d	f
Total	g	h	n

Quick formula

If the various numbers in the contingency table are represented by the letters shown in Table 13.2 then a quicker formula for calculating chi-squared on a 2×2 table is:

$$\chi^2 = \frac{n(ad-bc)^2}{efgh} = \frac{460 \times (20 \times 140 - 80 \times 220)^2}{100 \times 360 \times 240 \times 220} = 53.01$$

which apart from rounding error is the same as obtained above. With the **continuity correction** the quick formula becomes:

$$\chi^2 = \frac{n(|ad-bc| - n/2)^2}{efgh}, \quad \text{d.f.} = 1$$

In the example:

$$\chi^2 = \frac{460 \times (14800 - 230)^2}{100 \times 360 \times 240 \times 220} = 51.37$$

which again, apart from rounding error, is the same as obtained above.

Larger tables

The chi-squared test can also be applied to larger tables, generally called $\boldsymbol{r \times c}$ **tables**, where r denotes the number of rows in the table and c the number of columns.

$$\chi^2 = \Sigma \frac{(O-E)^2}{E}, \quad \text{d.f.} = (r-1) \times (c-1)$$

There is *no* continuity correction or exact test for contingency tables larger than 2×2. Cochran (1954) recommends that the approximation of the chi-squared test is valid provided less than 20% of the *expected* numbers are under 5 and none is less than 1. This restriction can sometimes be overcome by combining rows (or columns) with low expected numbers.

There is no quick formula for a general $r \times c$ table. (The special case of a $2 \times c$ or $r \times 2$ table is considered in the next section.) The expected numbers must be computed for each cell. The reasoning employed is the same as that described above for the 2×2 table. The general rule for calculating an expected number is:

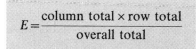

$$E = \frac{\text{column total} \times \text{row total}}{\text{overall total}}$$

It is worth pointing out that the chi-squared test is only valid if applied to the actual numbers in the various categories. It must never be applied to tables showing just proportions or percentages.

Example 13.1

Table 13.3(a) shows the results from a survey to compare the principal water sources in three villages in West Africa. The numbers and percentages of households using a river, a pond, or a spring are given. For example, in village A, 40.0% of households use mainly a river, 36.0% a pond and 24.0% a spring. *The calculation of such percentages is essential in interpreting contingency table data.* Overall, 70 of the 150 households use a river. If there were no difference between villages one would expect this same proportion of river usage in each village. Thus the expected numbers of households using a river are:

$$\frac{70}{150} \times 50 = 23.3, \quad \frac{70}{150} \times 60 = 28.0 \text{ and } \frac{70}{150} \times 40 = 18.7$$

The expected numbers can also be found by applying the general rule. For

Table 13.3 Comparison of principal sources of water used by households in three villages in West Africa.

(a) Observed numbers.

Water source	Village A	Village B	Village C	Total
River	20 (40.0%)	32 (53.3%)	18 (45.0%)	70 (46.7%)
Pond	18 (36.0%)	20 (33.3%)	12 (30.0%)	50 (33.3%)
Spring	12 (24.0%)	8 (13.3%)	10 (25.0%)	30 (20.0%)
Total	50 (100.0%)	60 (100.0%)	40 (100.0%)	150 (100.0%)

(b) Expected numbers.

Water source	Village A	Village B	Village C	Total
River	23.3	28.0	18.7	70
Pond	16.7	20.0	13.3	50
Spring	10.0	12.0	8.0	30
Total	50	60	40	150

example, the expected number of households using a river in village B is:

$$\frac{\text{row total (river)} \times \text{column total (B)}}{\text{overall total}} = \frac{70 \times 60}{150} = 28.0$$

The expected numbers for the whole table are given in Table 13.3(b).

$$\chi^2 = \Sigma \frac{(O-E)^2}{E}$$

$$= (20-23.3)^2/23.3 + (32-28.0)^2/28.0 + (18-18.7)^2/18.7 +$$
$$(18-16.7)^2/16.7 + (20-20.0)^2/20.0 + (12-13.3)^2/13.3 +$$
$$(12-10.0)^2/10.0 + (8-12.0)^2/12.0 + (10-8.0)^2/8.0$$
$$= 3.53$$

$$\text{d.f.} = (r-1) \times (c-1) = 2 \times 2 = 4$$

Since 3.53 is smaller than 5.39 (the 25% point of χ^2 with 4 d.f.), it is concluded that there is no significant difference between the villages in the percentages of households using different water sources ($P > 0.25$).

Shorter formula for 2 × c tables

A chi-squared test applied to a $2 \times c$ table, that is a table which has just two rows, gives an assessment of differences between the c proportions represented by the c columns of the table. A more compact formula is available in this case.

$$\chi^2 = \frac{N^2[\Sigma(r^2/n) - R^2/N]}{R(N-R)}, \quad \text{d.f.} = c - 1$$

n represents the total for a typical column and r the entry in the top row for that column. r^2/n is calculated for each column of the table and the results summed to give $\Sigma(r^2/n)$. N is the overall total and R the total of the top row. (For a table arranged with two *columns* rather than two rows, the words 'row' and 'column' should be interchanged in the above.)

Table 13.4 Prevalence of *Schistosoma mansoni* by occupation.

	Occupation				
S. mansoni	Fishermen	Farmers	Traders	Craftsmen	Total
Positive	22 (62.9%)	21 (48.8%)	17 (29.3%)	15 (51.7%)	75 (45.5%)
Negative	13	22	41	14	90
Total	35	43	58	29	165

Example 13.2
Table 13.4 shows the results of a survey in a rural area in central Africa to compare the prevalences of infection with *Schistosoma mansoni* among different occupations. Applying the shorter formula for χ^2 gives:

$$\Sigma(r^2/n) = 22^2/35 + 21^2/43 + 17^2/58 + 15^2/29$$
$$= 13.83 + 10.26 + 4.98 + 7.76 = 36.83$$

$$R^2/N = 75^2/165 = 34.09$$

$$\chi^2 = \frac{165^2(36.83 - 34.09)}{75 \times 90} = 11.05, \quad \text{d.f.} = 3$$

This is significant at the 2.5% level, suggesting that there may be an association between risk of infection and occupation, the prevalence of *S. mansoni* being higher among fishermen and lower among traders than among craftsmen and traders.

CHAPTER 14

Further Methods for Contingency Tables

Introduction

The analysis of contingency tables was introduced in Chapter 13 and the chi-squared test described. In this chapter we describe the methods to be used when this simple chi-squared test is either not appropriate or does not yield a sufficient analysis of the data. The first category includes cases when the sample size is too small for the chi-squared approximation to hold or when the proportions to be compared are paired (*see*, for example, Table 14.3). The second category includes the combined analysis of several contingency tables and the search for an increasing (or decreasing) trend over a $2 \times c$ table of proportions.

Exact test for 2 × 2 tables

As discussed in Chapter 13, the approximation of the chi-squared and normal tests for a 2×2 table may not be valid if the sample sizes are small. Cochran (1954) recommends the use of the alternative **exact test**, sometimes called Fisher's exact test, when:

(i) The overall total of the table is less than 20, or

(ii) The overall total is between 20 and 40 and the smallest of the four *expected* numbers is less than 5.

The test is most easily described in the context of a particular example. Table 14.1 shows the results from a study to compare two treatment regimes for controlling bleeding in haemophiliacs undergoing surgery. Only one (8%) of

Table 14.1 Comparison of two treatment regimes for controlling bleeding in haemophiliacs undergoing surgery.

Bleeding complications	Treatment regime A	Treatment regime B	Total
Yes	1	3	4
No	12	9	21
Total	13	12	25

the 13 haemophiliacs given treatment regime A suffered bleeding complications, compared to three out of 12 (25%) given regime B. These numbers are too small for the chi-squared test to be valid; the overall total, 25, is less than 40, and the smallest expected value, 1.9 (complications with regime B), is less than 5. The exact test is therefore indicated.

The exact test is based on calculating the exact probabilities of the observed table and of more 'extreme' tables with the same row and column totals, using the following formula.

$$\text{Exact probability of } 2 \times 2 \text{ table} = \frac{e!\ f!\ g!\ h!}{n!\ a!\ b!\ c!\ d!}$$

where the notation is the same as that defined in Table 13.2. The exclamation mark denotes the factorial of the number and means all the integers from the number down to 1 multiplied together. (0! is defined to equal 1.) Many calculators have a key for factorial, although this expression may be easily computed by cancelling factors in the top and bottom. The exact probability of Table 14.1 is therefore:

$$\frac{4!\ 21!\ 13!\ 12!}{25!\ 1!\ 3!\ 12!\ 9!} = \frac{4 \times 13 \times 12 \times 11 \times 10}{25 \times 24 \times 23 \times 22} = 0.2261$$

(21! being cancelled into 25!, for example, leaving $25 \times 24 \times 23 \times 22$).

In order to test the null hypothesis that there is no difference between the treatment regimes, we need to calculate not only the probability of the observed table but also the probability that a more extreme table could occur by chance. Altogether there are five possible tables which have the same row and column totals as the data. These are shown in Table 14.2 together with their probabilities, which total 1. The observed case is Table 14.2(b) with a probability of 0.2261. Defining more extreme as less probable, more extreme tables are 14.2(a) and 14.2(e) with probabilities 0.0391 and 0.0565 respectively. The total probability needed for the significance level is therefore $0.2261 + 0.0391 + 0.0565 = 0.3217$, and so the difference between the regimes is clearly not significant.

$$\text{Significance level (approach I)} = \text{probability of observed table} + \text{probability of less probable tables}$$

An alternative approach is to restrict the calculation to extreme tables showing differences in the *same* direction as that observed, and then to double the resulting probability in order to cover differences in the other direction.

Table 14.2 All possible tables with the same row and column totals as Table 14.1, together with their probabilities.

(a)

0	4	4
13	8	21
13	12	25

$p = 0.0391$

(b)

1	3	4
12	9	21
13	12	25

$p = 0.2261$

(c)

2	2	4
11	10	21
13	12	25

$p = 0.4070$

(d)

3	1	4
10	11	21
13	12	25

$p = 0.2713$

(e)

4	0	4
9	12	21
13	12	25

$p = 0.0565$

In this example, the significance level thus obtained would be twice the sum of the probabilities of Tables 14.2(a) and 14.2(b), namely $2 \times (0.0391 + 0.2261) = 0.5304$. Neither method is clearly superior to the other, but the second method is simpler to carry out. Although the two approaches give different results, the choice is unlikely, in practice, to affect the assessment of whether the observed difference is due to chance or to a real effect.

$$\text{Significance level (approach II)} = 2 \times \left[\begin{array}{c}\text{probability of observed table} + \\ \text{more extreme tables in same direction}\end{array}\right]$$

Comparison of two proportions—paired case

In some studies we are interested in comparing two proportions calculated from observations which are paired in some way. This arises whenever the two proportions are measured on the *same* individuals (*see* following example) or from case–control studies and clinical trials in which a **matched paired design** has been used (*see* Chapters 24 and 25 respectively).

For example, consider the results of an experiment to compare the Bell and Kato–Katz methods for detecting *Schistosoma mansoni* eggs in faeces in which two subsamples from each of 315 specimens were analysed, one by each method. The results are arranged in a 2 × 2 contingency table in Table 14.3(a), showing the agreement between the two methods. It is not this agreement, however, that we are concerned with here. We are interested primarily in comparing the proportions of specimens found positive with the two methods. These were 238/315 (75.6%) using the Bell method and 198/315 (62.9%) using the Kato–Katz method. Note that it would be incorrect to arrange the data as in Table 14.3(b) and to apply the standard chi-squared test, as this would take no account of the *paired* nature of the data, namely that it was the *same* 315 specimens examined with each method, and not 630 different ones.

Table 14.3 Comparison of Bell and Kato–Katz methods for detecting *Schistosoma mansoni* eggs in faeces. The same 315 specimens were examined using each method. Data from Sleigh *et al.* (1982) *Transactions of the Royal Society of Tropical Medicine and Hygiene* **76**, 403–6 (with permission)

(a) Correct layout.

		Kato–Katz		
		+	−	Total
Bell	+	184	54	238
	−	14	63	77
Total		198	117	315

(b) Incorrect layout.

Result	Bell	Kato–Katz	Total
+	238	198	436
−	77	117	194
Total	315	315	630

The correct approach is as follows. One hundred and eighty-four specimens were positive with both methods and 63 were negative with both. These 247 specimens therefore give us no information about which of the two methods is better at detecting *S. mansoni* eggs. The information we require is entirely contained in the 68 specimens for which the methods did not agree. Of these 54 were positive with the Bell method only compared to 14 positive with the Kato–Katz method only.

If there was no difference in the abilities of the methods to detect *S. mansoni* eggs, we would not of course expect complete agreement since different subsamples were examined, but we would expect on average half the disagreements to be positive with the Bell method only and half to be positive with the Kato–Katz method only. Thus an appropriate significance test is to compare the proportion found positive with the Bell method only, namely 54/68, with the hypothetical value of 0.5. This may be done using the normal test (with continuity correction), as described in Chapter 12. This gives:

$$z = \frac{|54/68 - 0.5| - 1/(2 \times 68)}{\sqrt{(0.5 \times 0.5/68)}} = 4.73$$

indicating that the Bell method is significantly better ($P < 0.001$) than the Kato–Katz method at detecting *S. mansoni* eggs. (Note that exactly the same result would have been obtained had the proportion positive with the Kato–Katz method only, namely 14/68, been compared with 0.5.)

McNemar's chi-squared test

There is also an alternative chi-squared test, called **McNemar's chi-squared test**, which is based on the numbers of **discordant pairs**, r and s. The version including a *continuity correction* is:

$$\chi^2_{\text{paired}} = \frac{(|r - s| - 1)^2}{r + s}, \quad \text{d.f.} = 1$$

In the example $r = 54$ and $s = 14$, giving:

$$\chi^2 = \frac{(|54 - 14| - 1)^2}{54 + 14} = \frac{39^2}{68} = 22.36, \quad \text{d.f.} = 1, \quad P < 0.001$$

Apart from rounding error, this χ^2 value is the same as the square of the z value obtained above ($4.73^2 = 22.37$), the two tests being mathematically equivalent.

Validity

The use of McNemar's chi-squared test or the equivalent normal test is valid provided that the total number of discordant pairs is at least 10. If there are less than 10 discordant pairs, exact binomial probabilities must be calculated, as described in Chapter 12.

Confidence interval

The proportion of specimens found positive with the Bell method was 0.7556 compared to 0.6286 with the Kato–Katz method. The difference between the proportions was therefore 0.1270. This difference, together with its standard error, can also be calculated from the numbers of discordant pairs, r and s, and the total number of pairs, n.

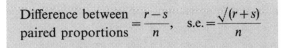

$$\text{Difference between paired proportions} = \frac{r-s}{n}, \quad \text{s.e.} = \frac{\sqrt{(r+s)}}{n}$$

Here this gives a difference, $(r-s)/n = 40/315 = 0.1270$, the same as calculated directly from the proportions, with s.e. $= (\sqrt{68})/315 = 0.0262$. An approximate confidence interval may be based on the normal distribution.

$$\text{c.i.} = \frac{(r-s)}{n} \pm z' \frac{\sqrt{(r+s)}}{n}$$

The 95% confidence interval for the difference between the proportions of specimens found positive with the Bell and Kato–Katz methods is therefore:

$$0.1270 \pm 1.96 \times 0.0262 = 0.0756,\ 0.1784$$

This means a positivity rate between 7.6% and 17.8% higher if the Bell method is used to detect *S. mansoni* eggs than if the Kato–Katz method is used.

Analysing several 2 × 2 tables

A very important general point to realize when carrying out an analysis is that it may be misleading to pool dissimilar subsets of the data. For example, consider the hypothetical results, shown in Table 14.4, from a survey carried out to compare the prevalence of antibodies to leptospirosis in rural and urban areas of the West Indies. The main point to notice is that, for both males and females, the prevalence is higher in rural areas, but that when the sexes are combined there appears to be no difference. This is caused by a combination of two factors:

(i) The prevalence of antibodies is not the same for males and females. It is much lower among females in both areas.

(ii) The samples from the rural and urban areas have different sex compositions. The proportion of males is 100/200 (50%) in the urban sample but only 50/200 (25%) in the rural sample.

Sex is said to be a **confounding** variable because it is related both to the variable of interest (prevalence of antibodies) and to the groups being compared (rural and urban). Ignoring sex in the analysis leads to a **bias** in the

Table 14.4 Comparison of prevalence of antibodies to leptospirosis between rural and urban areas.

(a) Males.

Antibodies	Rural	Urban	Total
Yes	36 (72%)	50 (50%)	86
No	14	50	64
Total	50	100	150

$\chi^2 = 5.73$, d.f. = 1, $P < 0.025$

(b) Females.

Antibodies	Rural	Urban	Total
Yes	24 (16%)	10 (10%)	34
No	126	90	216
Total	150	100	250

$\chi^2 = 1.36$, d.f. = 1, $P \simeq 0.25$

(c) Males and females combined.

Antibodies	Rural	Urban	Total
Yes	60 (30%)	60 (30%)	120
No	140	140	280
Total	200	200	400

results. It is therefore important to analyse males and females separately. Applying the chi-squared test shows that the difference between the rural and urban areas is significant for males but not for females (Table 14.4). A summary test combining these two pieces of information is described below, and methods of standardization to adjust the overall proportions to reflect the sex differences are described in Chapter 15.

In this instance pooling the sexes masked a difference that existed. In other situations pooling dissimilar subsets of the data could suggest a difference or association where none exists, or could even suggest a difference the opposite way around to one which does exist. Another example is in the assessment of whether persons suffering from schistosomiasis have a higher mortality rate than uninfected persons. In this case it would be important to take age into account since both the risk of dying and the risk of having schistosomiasis increase with age. If age were not allowed for, schistosomiasis would appear to be associated with increased mortality, even if it were not, as those with schistosomiasis would be on average older and therefore more likely to die than younger uninfected persons.

Mantel–Haenszel chi-squared test

When confounding is present, it is important to analyse the relevant subsets of the data separately. It is often useful, however, to apply a summary test which pools the evidence from the individual subsets but which takes account of the confounding factor(s). This is particularly true when a difference is present but not significant in the individual subsets, maybe because of their small sample size. The Mantel–Haenszel chi-squared test is used for this purpose when the data consist of several 2×2 tables. The following three values are calculated from each table and then summed over the tables (the notation is as defined in Table 13.2):

(i) The observed value, a,
(ii) The expected value for a, $E_a = eg/n$, and
(iii) The variance of a, $V_a = efgh/[n^2(n-1)]$.

The chi-squared value (with *continuity correction*) is:

$$\chi^2_{\text{MH}} = \frac{(|\Sigma a - \Sigma E_a| - 0.5)^2}{\Sigma V_a}, \quad \text{d.f.} = 1$$

Note that it has just 1 degree of freedom irrespective of how many tables are summarized.

The calculations for the data presented in Table 14.4 are laid out in Table 14.5(a). A total of 60 persons in the rural area had antibodies to leptospirosis compared with an expected number of 49.1, based on assuming no difference in prevalence between rural and urban areas. The Mantel–Haenszel χ^2 value equals 7.08 and is significant at the 1% level.

It may seem strange that this test appears to be based entirely on the observed and expected values of a and not also on the other cells in the tables. This is not really the case, however, since once the value of a is known the values of b, c and d can be calculated from the totals of the table. If the Mantel–Haenszel test is applied to a single 2×2 table, the χ^2 value obtained is close to, but not exactly equal to, the standard χ^2 value. It is slightly smaller, equalling $(n-1)/n$ times the standard value. This difference is negligible for values of n of 20 or more, as required for the validity of the chi-squared test.

Table 14.5 Calculation of Mantel–Haenszel χ^2 test, applied to data in Table 14.4.

(a) The test.

Subset	a	E_a	V_a
Males	36	28.7	$86\times 64\times 50\times 100/(150^2\times 149)=8.2088$
Females	24	20.4	$34\times 216\times 150\times 100/(250^2\times 249)=7.0786$
Total	60	49.1	15.2874

$$\chi^2=\frac{(|60-49.1|-0.5)^2}{15.2874}=\frac{10.4^2}{15.2874}=7.08,\ \text{d.f.}=1,\ P<0.01$$

(b) Rule of 5, to check validity.

Subset	Min (e,g)	$g-f$	Max $(0,g-f)$
Males	50	−14	0
Females	34	−66	0
Total	84		0

Validity

The Mantel–Haenszel χ^2 test is an approximation. Its adequacy is assessed by the 'rule of 5'. Two additional values are calculated for each table and summed over the tables. These are:

(i) Min (e, g), that is the smaller of e and g, and

(ii) Max $(0, g-f)$, which equals 0 if g is smaller than or equal to f, and $g-f$ if g is larger.

Both sums must differ from the total of the expected values, ΣE_a, by at least 5 for the test to be valid. The details of these calculations for the leptospirosis data are shown in Table 14.5(b). The two sums, 84 and zero, both differ from 49.1 by 5 or more, validating the use of the Mantel–Haenszel χ^2 test.

Chi-squared test for trend

The standard chi-squared test for a $2\times c$ table is a general test to assess whether there are differences among the c proportions. When the categories in the columns have a natural order, however, a more sensitive test is to look for an increasing (or decreasing) trend in the proportions over the columns. An example is given in Table 14.6, which shows data from a study

Table 14.6 Relationship between triceps skinfold and early menarche. Data from a study on obesity in women—Beckles *et al.* (1985), *International Journal of Obesity* **9**, 127–35.

	Triceps skinfold group			
Age at menarche	Small	Intermediate	Large	Total
< 12 years	15 (8.8%)	29 (12.8%)	36 (19.4%)	80
12 + years	156	197	150	503
Total	171	226	186	583
Score for trend test	1	2	3	

on obesity in women. It can be seen that the proportion of women who had experienced early menarche increased with triceps skinfold size. This trend can be tested using the **chi-squared test for trend**, which has 1 degree of freedom.

The first step is to assign **scores** to the columns to describe the shape of the trend. The usual choice is simply to number the columns 1, 2, 3, etc., as shown here (or equivalently 0, 1, 2, etc.). This represents a trend that goes up (or down) in equal steps from column to column, and is adequate for most circumstances. Another possibility would have been to use the means of the triceps skinfold measurements in each group, reflecting a linear trend with absolute value of triceps skinfold. (Note that the difference between the standard χ^2 value and the trend test χ^2 value provides a chi-squared value with $(c-2)$ degrees of freedom to test for **departures from the fitted trend**.)

The next step is to calculate three quantities for each column of the table and to sum the results of each. These are:

(i) rx, the product of the entry, r, in the top row of the column and the score, x,

(ii) nx, the product of the total, n, of the column and the score, x, and

(iii) nx^2, the product of the total, n, of the column and the square of the score, x^2.

Using N to denote the overall total and R the total of the top row, the formula for the chi-squared test for trend (with continuity correction) is:

$$\chi^2_{\text{trend}} = \frac{(|A|-0.5)^2}{B}, \quad \text{d.f.}=1$$

where $A = \Sigma(rx) - \dfrac{R}{N}\Sigma(nx)$ and $B = \dfrac{R(N-R)}{N^2(N-1)}[N\,\Sigma(nx^2) - (\Sigma nx)^2]$

There are various different forms for this test, most of which are algebraically equivalent. The only difference is that in some forms $(N-1)$ is replaced by N in the calculation of B. This difference is unimportant. The form chosen here is both relatively simple to apply and easily extended to several $2 \times c$ tables (*see below*). *The subtraction of 0.5 in the top row is the continuity correction. This should be omitted if the scores are not simply the column numbers.*

The calculations for the data presented in Table 14.6 are as follows:

$$\Sigma(rx) = 15 \times 1 + 29 \times 2 + 36 \times 3 = 181$$

$$\Sigma(nx) = 171 \times 1 + 226 \times 2 + 186 \times 3 = 1181$$

$$\Sigma(nx^2) = 171 \times 1 + 226 \times 4 + 186 \times 9 = 2749$$

$$R = 80, \; N = 583, \; N - R = 503$$

$$A = 181 - \frac{80}{583} \times 1181 = 18.9417$$

$$B = \frac{80 \times 503}{583^2 \times 582} \times (583 \times 2749 - 1181^2) = 42.2927$$

$$\chi^2 = \frac{(18.9417 - 0.5)^2}{42.2927} = 8.04, \quad \text{d.f.} = 1, \quad P < 0.005$$

Thus the trend of an increasing proportion of women who had experienced early menarche with increasing triceps skinfold size is highly significant ($P < 0.005$).

Extension for several 2 × c tables

When the data consist of several subsets which cannot be pooled because of confounding variables, any trend tests should be carried out on each subset. A summary test is also available, however, which combines the evidence from the separate trends taking into account the confounding. This is a chi-squared test, which has 1 degree of freedom, irrespective of the number of subsets. A and B are calculated for each of the individual tables as described above and then summed. The χ^2 value is:

$$\text{Summary } \chi^2_{\text{trend}} = \frac{(|\Sigma A| - 0.5)^2}{\Sigma B}, \quad \text{d.f.} = 1$$

More complex techniques

Two complex techniques will be briefly mentioned as they are powerful methods for analysing proportions and contingency tables. The first is **logistic regression**, a method for analysing proportions analogous to multiple regression for continuous variables. The analysis of several 2×2 (or $2 \times c$) tables can be considered as a special case of this. For example, the data in Table 14.4 show how the prevalence of antibodies to leptospirosis varies with respect to two factors, sex and type of area. Logistic regression is more general than the chi-squared methods described above since it allows both the inclusion of *continuous* explanatory variables and the assessment of *interaction* (*see* Chapter 8) between the variables. Logistic regression is so called because it investigates the linear dependence of the **logistic transformation** of the proportion on several explanatory variables, where the logistic transformation, or **logit** for short, is defined as:

$$\text{Logit} = \log_e \left[\frac{\text{proportion}}{1 - \text{proportion}} \right]$$

The model is fitted using a mathematical technique called **maximum likelihood**, which also takes account of the fact that the variation of a proportion has a binomial distribution.

A second and similar technique is the use of **log linear models**. Both methods can be carried out using the computer package GLIM (1978), whose name is an acronym for generalized linear interactive modelling. A series of different models is fitted, as in multiple regression. The significance of a particular variable is assessed by fitting two models, one including and the other excluding that variable. The test is based on the *difference* of the **deviances** (the equivalent to the residual sum of squares, *see* Chapter 10) of the two models. This difference is distributed as χ^2, with degrees of freedom equal to the number of extra parameters fitted. For more details see Anderson *et al.* (1980), or for a mathematical approach see Dobson (1984).

Good descriptions of logistic regression can also be found in the books by Breslow and Day (1980), and Schlesselman (1982). Although these were both written in the context of case–control studies (*see* Chapter 24), the methods apply more generally to the analysis of proportions. These books also contain descriptions of **conditional logistic regression**. This is the version of logistic regression appropriate for the analysis of *matched* data, which can be considered as a multivariate extension of McNemar's paired χ^2 test.

CHAPTER 15

Measures of Mortality and Morbidity

Introduction

We now turn to the measure of mortality and morbidity and consider in particular the use of rates, a mortality or morbidity rate being the number of persons dying or falling ill within a given period of time divided by the total number of persons in whom such an event might have been observed. Definitions of the commonly used rates will be given first. The problem of calculating and comparing rates for study populations which may have differing age–sex compositions will then be considered, and the statistical techniques of standardization of rates will be described. Finally, methods of analysis will be briefly reviewed.

Birth and death rates

Population birth and death rates are based on statistics collected over a calendar year. For convenience, these rates are usually multiplied by 1000 to avoid small decimal numbers and expressed as, for example, the number of births per 1000 members of the population per year. The common measures are:

1* Birth rate $= \dfrac{\text{number of births in year}}{\text{mid-year population}} \times 1000$

2* Fertility rate $= \dfrac{\text{number of livebirths in year}}{\text{mid-year population of women aged 15–44}} \times 1000$

3* Crude mortality rate $= \dfrac{\text{number of deaths in year}}{\text{mid-year population}} \times 1000$

4* Age- (sex-) specific mortality rate =

$$\frac{\text{number of deaths during year in particular age (sex) group}}{\text{mid-year population of age (sex) group}} \times 1000$$

5† Infant mortality rate =

$$\frac{\text{number of deaths in year under 1 year of age}}{\text{number of livebirths in year}} \times 1000$$

6† Neonatal mortality rate =

$$\frac{\text{number of deaths in year under 28 days of age}}{\text{number of livebirths in year}} \times 1000$$

7† Perinatal mortality rate =

$$\frac{\text{number of stillbirths} + \text{deaths under 7 days of age in year}}{\text{total number of births (live} + \text{still) in year}} \times 1000$$

8* Cause-specific mortality rate =

$$\frac{\text{number of deaths in year due to a particular cause}}{\text{mid-year population}} \times 1000$$

9† Proportional mortality rate (expressed as a percentage) =

$$\frac{\text{number of deaths in year due to a particular cause}}{\text{total number of deaths in year}} \times 100$$

10† Case fatality rate (expressed as a percentage) =

$$\frac{\text{number of deaths in year due to a particular disease}}{\text{number of cases of that disease}} \times 100$$

Note that although these measures are all called 'rates', they are in fact of two distinct types. Those marked with an asterisk (*), numbers 1, 2, 3, 4, and 8, are the only ones that are truly **rates** in the mathematical sense of measuring how rapidly some attribute of a population changes with time. Thus, for example, the birth rate measures how fast the size of a population is increasing due to new births, and the crude death rate measures how fast it is decreasing due to deaths. The other measures, those marked with a dagger (†), numbers 5, 6, 7, 9, and 10, are more correctly termed **risks**, as they are the probabilities of occurrence of certain events. Thus, the case fatality rate measures the risk that a person, having contracted a particular disease, will die from it. Although the distinction between risks and rates was clearly described by William Farr in the early nineteenth century, it is only in recent years that it has again attracted attention (Vandenbrouke 1985) and current terminology remains muddled. The difference is discussed again later in the chapter in the context of measuring incidence of disease.

Note also that an indirect form of calculation is used for some of the risk-type measures. For example, the infant mortality rate is the risk that a child will die before its first birthday. The direct way to measure this would be to follow a cohort of births and record the proportion of children in that cohort who die before their first birthday. For convenience, however, the infant mortality rate is estimated by the ratio of the number of deaths under one year of age to the number of livebirths in the year. The numerator will therefore include some deaths among children who were born the previous year and, correspondingly, miss some infant deaths among children born during the current year which do not occur until the following year. In a stable population it is assumed that these two factors will cancel each other out. A similar consideration applies to the estimation of neonatal and perinatal mortality rates.

Measuring mortality in a research study

The definitions of mortality rates given above were based on the number of deaths occurring during a calendar year divided by the mid-year population. In research studies, however, not only may mortality be measured over periods other than 1 year, but also people may be followed for differing lengths of time due to a variety of reasons. These reasons may include the gradual recruitment of study subjects in order to spread the workload over time, the recruitment of newborns or new cases of disease as they arise, the recruitment of new migrants into the area, and the loss to follow-up of individuals due to their migration out of the area, withdrawal of willingness to participate, or death. The number of deaths observed is therefore related to the total number of **person–years of observation**, rather than to a mid-year population. Note that one person–year of observation may result from one person being observed for a whole year or, for example, from 12 persons being observed for just one month each.

$$\text{Mortality rate} = \frac{\text{number of deaths}}{\text{person–years of observation}} \times 1000$$

The mortality rate is usually multiplied by 1000 and the result expressed per 1000 person–years of follow-up. When reporting rates, it is important to make the distinction between per 1000 per year, which implies a group of persons all followed for the same length of time, and per 1000 person–years.

Consider the common situation where mortality is measured by surveying a community twice and counting the number of persons who died in the intervening period. A person seen at both surveys contributes the number of years between the surveys to the total person–years of observation. A person who died or moved in the intervening period contributes the number of years between the first survey and the date of death or migration, while an individual who was born or moved into the community between the surveys contributes the number of years between the date of birth or of joining the community and the second survey. If the exact date of death or movement cannot be determined it is usually assumed to have occurred half-way through the interval between the surveys.

Measures of morbidity

There are two principal measures of the disease experience of a community. The **incidence** is the number of *new cases* of a disease during a specified period of time related to the number of *persons at risk* of contracting the disease; while the **prevalence** is based on the total number of *existing cases* among the *whole population*. The size of the prevalence depends on both the size of the incidence and the duration of the disease; for a given size of incidence the prevalence will be much greater for a disease which lasts years than for a disease which lasts only a few days.

Prevalence

Prevalence may be measured either at a single point in time (**point prevalence**) or over a period of time (**period prevalence**). It is usually expressed as a percentage or, when very small, as per 1000 population.

$$\textbf{1}\ \text{(Point) prevalence rate} = \frac{\text{number of persons with disease at a particular point in time}}{\text{total population}}$$

$$\textbf{2}\ \text{Period prevalence rate} = \frac{\text{total number of persons with disease at some time during specified period}}{\text{total population at mid-point of interval}}$$

The point prevalence is the more common and more useful measure, and is usually referred to simply as the prevalence.

Incidence

There are two conceptually different ways of defining incidence; it may be measured either as a risk or as a rate. The **incidence risk** is the probability that a person initially free from the disease develops it at some time during the period of observation. It is usually expressed as a percentage or, if small, as per 1000 persons. The **incidence rate**, on the other hand, is the rate of contracting the disease among those still at risk—when a person contracts the disease, they are no longer at risk. The number of new cases is related not to those initially at risk but to the *average* number at risk during the period, multiplied by the length of the period, or equivalently to the total number of **person–years at risk** (pyar) during the period. It is usually multiplied by 1000 and expressed per 1000 person–years at risk. For a common disease, such as diarrhoea, which may attack more than once, the incidence rate measures the average number of attacks per person per year (at risk).

$$\textbf{1}\ \text{Incidence risk} = \frac{\text{number of new cases of disease in a specified period of time}}{\text{number at risk of contracting disease at beginning of period}}$$

$$\textbf{2}\ \text{Incidence rate} = \frac{\text{number of new cases of disease in a specified period of time}}{\text{number of person years at risk during period (average number at risk of contracting disease during period} \times \text{length of the period)}}$$

Person–years at risk is calculated in a similar way to that described above for person–years of observation. The only difference is for diseases which may occur more than once, when a person contributes the total length of time free from the disease during the study, rather than just the time from the start of the study to first contracting the disease.

For a **rare disease**, such as many cancers, the two measures of incidence are basically the same, since the number at risk will approximately equal the total population at all times. For this reason they are often not clearly distinguished. For a **common disease**, however, the risk and rate are different.

For example, consider measles during the second year of life in a country where there is little measles immunization. Suppose that 1000 previously uninfected children are followed from their first birthday for one year and that 140 develop measles, leaving 860 still at risk at the end of the year. The incidence risk is then the probability that a child who had escaped measles during the first year of life contracts it during the second and equals 140/1000 =0.1400 or 14.0%. The incidence rate, on the other hand, is the rate of contracting measles during the second year of life. If we assume that the cases of measles are evenly spread throughout the year, the average number at risk equals the average of those at risk at the beginning and at the end of the year, that is (1000 + 860)/2 or 930. The incidence rate therefore equals 140/930 = 0.1505 or 150.5 per 1000 child–years at risk.

Relative risk

The comparison of two incidences is sometimes summarized by their ratio rather than their difference. For example, children of smokers may be found to be three times more likely to develop asthma than children of non-smokers. This ratio is called the **relative risk** and is described more fully in Chapter 24.

Standardized rates

Since both the risk of dying and the risk of contracting most diseases are related to age, and since they often differ for the two sexes, the crude mortality rate and overall incidence and prevalence rates depend critically on the age–sex composition of the population. For example, a relatively older population would have a higher crude mortality rate than a younger population even if, age for age, the mortalities were the same. It is therefore misleading to use these overall rates when comparing two different populations unless they have the same age–sex structure. Instead the comparison should be based on the individual age–sex specific rates with the overall test of any difference being carried out by the Mantel–Haenszel χ^2 test applied to the separate age–sex groups (*see* Chapter 14).

It is also useful, however, to have overall summary rates that are adjusted for any age–sex differences. This is achieved by the use of a standard population with the methods of direct or indirect standardization. In the **direct method** the age–sex specific rates from each of the populations under study are applied to a standard population to give **age–sex adjusted mortality (or morbidity) rates**, while in the **indirect method** the age–sex specific rates from a standard population are applied to each of the populations of interest to give **standardized mortality (or morbidity) ratios** (which in turn may be used to give adjusted rates). This comparison is summarized in Table 15.1 which also shows the different data required by the two approaches.

The choice of method is usually governed by the availability of data and by their (relative) accuracy. For example, in comparing mortality rates from different countries, the indirect method will be preferable if it is difficult to obtain national data on age–sex specific mortality rates. In general, indirect standardization is more commonly employed for mortalities and incidences, and direct standardization for prevalences.

Table 15.1 Comparison of direct and indirect methods of standardization.

	Direct standardization	Indirect standardization
Data required		
Study population(s)	Age–sex specific rates	Age–sex composition + total deaths (or cases)
Standard population	Age–sex composition	Age–sex specific rates (+ overall rate)
Method	Study rates applied to standard population	Standard rates applied to study population
Result	Age–sex adjusted rate	Standardized mortality (morbidity) ratio (+ age–sex adjusted rate)

Both methods can be extended to adjust for other factors besides age and sex, such as different ethnic compositions of the study groups. The direct method can also be used to calculate **standardized means**, such as age–sex adjusted mean blood pressure levels for different occupational groups.

The techniques of direct and indirect standardization will be described by considering two examples relating to the epidemiology of onchocerciasis, a parasitic disease which, in its severest form, leads to blindness.

Direct standardization

Table 15.2 shows the age–sex specific prevalences and overall crude prevalences of onchocerciasis in each of two villages, A and B. Note that the prevalence of onchocerciasis increases with age, that it is higher for males than for females, and also that the age–sex compositions of the samples from the two villages differ. The overall prevalences must therefore be adjusted for age and sex before they can meaningfully be compared. This will be done using the method of direct standardization.

First, a standard population is identified. This is usually one of the following: either one of the study populations, or the total of both populations (as will be described here), or the census population from the local area or country. The choice is to some extent arbitrary. It should be noted, however, that different choices lead to different summary rates but that this is unlikely to affect the interpretation of the results.

Second, the number of persons in the standard population that would be infected if the age–sex specific prevalence rates were the same as those in village A is calculated. For example, consider males aged 0–4 years. Two out of 36 in this group were infected in village A, giving a prevalence rate of 5.6%. There are 50 males of this age in the standard population, and if the

Table 15.2 Use of direct standardization to compare the prevalences of onchocerciasis in two villages, A and B. The total population examined in the two villages has been used as the standard.

	Village A			Village B			Standard population (villages A + B)		
Age (yrs)	Number examined	Number infected	Percentage infected	Number examined	Number infected	Percentage infected	Number examined	Number infected using rates from Village A	Number infected using rates from Village B
Males									
0–4	36	2	5.6	14	1	7.1	50	2.8	3.6
5–9	42	4	9.5	28	4	14.3	70	6.7	10.0
10–14	12	3	25.0	10	9	90.0	22	5.5	19.8
15–29	6	4	66.7	10	10	100.0	16	10.7	16.0
30–49	11	9	81.8	11	11	100.0	22	18.0	22.0
50+	21	17	81.0	8	8	100.0	29	23.5	29.0
Females									
0–4	35	1	2.9	17	1	5.9	52	1.5	3.1
5–9	52	4	7.7	15	2	13.3	67	5.2	8.9
10–14	15	3	20.0	9	4	44.4	24	4.8	10.7
15–29	24	14	58.3	12	11	91.7	36	21.0	33.0
30–49	25	19	76.0	17	17	100.0	42	31.9	42.0
50+	8	6	75.0	7	7	100.0	15	11.3	15.0
Total	287	86	30.0	158	85	53.8	445	142.9	213.1
Age–sex adjusted prevalence (%)								32.1	47.9

prevalence were also 5.6% this would mean that $2/36 \times 50 = 2.8$ of them would be infected. The numbers in the other age–sex groups are shown in Table 15.2. In total there would be 142.9 out of 445 persons suffering from onchocerciasis in the standard population, giving an overall prevalence rate of 32.1% ($142.9/445 \times 100$). This is called the **age–sex adjusted prevalence rate** for village A.

Age–sex adjusted prevalence rate	=	Overall prevalence rate in standard population if age–sex specific rates were the same as those of the population of interest

The age–sex adjusted prevalence rate for village B is calculated in the same way. It equals 47.9%, considerably higher than that for village A. The Mantel–Haenszel χ^2 test comparing the prevalence rates between these two villages is highly significant ($\chi^2 = 21.7$, d.f. = 1, $P < 0.001$).

Indirect standardization

Table 15.3 shows the results for mortality from a large study in an area endemic for onchocerciasis, in which 12 816 persons aged 30 years or more were followed for a year. One feature of interest was to assess whether blindness, the severest consequence of onchocerciasis, leads to an increased risk of dying. It is important to look at the individual age–sex mortality rates, since not only does mortality increase with age and differ slightly between the sexes but the prevalence of blindness also increases with age and is higher for males than for females. A blind population would therefore tend to be older and have a higher proportion of males, and consequently a higher crude mortality rate, than a non-blind population, even if the individual age–sex specific rates were the same. An overall comparison between the blind and non-blind will be obtained using the method of indirect standardization.

As for direct standardization, the first step is to identify a standard population. The usual choices are as before, with the restrictions that age–sex specific mortality rates are needed for the standard population and that the population chosen for this should therefore be large enough to have reliable estimates of these rates. In this example the rates among the non-blind will be used.

These standard rates are then applied to the population of interest to calculate the number of deaths that would have been expected in this population if the mortality experience was the same as that in the standard

Table 15.3 Use of indirect standardization to compare mortality rates between the blind and non-blind, collected as part of a one-year study in an area endemic for onchocerciasis. The mortality rates among the non-blind have been used as the standard rates.

	Non-blind persons			Blind persons				Expected number of deaths among blind if rates were the same as those of the non-blind
Age (yrs)	Number followed	Number deaths	Deaths/ 1000/yr	Number followed	Percentage blind	Number deaths	Deaths/ 1000/yr	
Males								
30–39	2400	19	7.9	120	4.8	3	25.0	0.95
40–49	1590	21	13.2	171	9.7	7	40.9	2.26
50–59	1120	20	17.9	244	17.9	13	53.3	4.36
60+	610	20	32.8	237	28.0	24	101.3	7.77
Females								
30–39	3100	23	7.4	84	2.6	2	23.8	0.62
40–49	1610	22	13.7	69	4.1	3	43.5	0.94
50–59	930	16	17.2	168	15.3	8	47.6	2.89
60+	270	8	29.6	93	25.6	9	96.8	2.76
Total	11630	149	12.8	1186	9.3	69	58.2	22.55
SMR			1.0				3.1 (69/22.5)	
Age–sex adjusted mortality rate			12.8				39.7 (3.1 × 12.8)	

population. For example, one would expect a proportion of 19/2400 of the 120 blind males aged 30–39 years to die, if their risk of dying was the same as that of the non-blind males of similar age. This gives an expected 0.95 deaths for this age group. In total, 22.55 deaths would have been expected among the blind compared to an observed number of 69. The ratio of the observed to the expected number of deaths is called the **standardized mortality ratio** (SMR). It equals 3.1 (69/22.55) in this case.

$$\text{Standardized mortality ratio (SMR)} = \frac{\text{observed number of deaths}}{\text{expected number of deaths if the age–sex specific rates were the same as those of the standard population}}$$

The SMR measures how much more (or less) likely a person is to die in the study population compared to someone of the same age and sex in the standard population. A value of 1 means that they are equally likely to die, a value larger than 1 that they are more likely to die, and a value smaller than 1 that they are less likely to do so. The SMR is sometimes multiplied by 100 and expressed as a percentage.

Since the non-blind population was used as the standard, its expected and observed numbers of deaths are equal resulting in an SMR of 1. Comparing the two SMRs indicates that, overall, blind persons were 3.1 times more likely to die during the year than non-blind persons. The Mantel–Haenszel χ^2 test is highly significant ($\chi^2 = 55.7$, d.f. $= 1$, $P < 0.001$).

Age–sex adjusted mortality rates may be obtained by multiplying the SMRs by the crude mortality rate of the standard population, when this is known. This gives age–sex adjusted mortality rates of 12.8 and 39.7/1000/year for the non-blind and blind populations respectively.

$$\text{Age–sex adjusted mortality rate} = \text{SMR} \times \text{crude mortality rate of standard population}$$

Analysis of rates

The methods described in Chapters 12, 13, and 14 relating to proportions apply to the analysis of prevalence rates and of those mortality and incidence measures that are risks, since these are simply proportions. These methods may also be applied to the analysis of those mortality and incidence measures that are rates, whenever the number of deaths (or new cases of disease) is small compared to the average number of persons at risk, as is often the case, the rate being treated as if it were a proportion. Alternatively, mortality and incidence rates may be analysed using the Poisson distribution, described in Chapter 17, and log linear models, mentioned in Chapter 14, provided that the deaths (or cases) are occurring independently of each other and randomly in time.

CHAPTER 16

Survival Analysis

Introduction

In Chapter 15 we considered how to measure and analyse mortality rates. In this chapter we describe the related methods of survival analysis, which focus not only on whether or not a person has died but also on the length of **survival time** before death. The methods of survival analysis can also be applied to events other than deaths, such as in a study of the duration of breast-feeding where the terminal event might be the completion of weaning.

Life tables

The survival pattern of a community is often displayed as a **life table**, which may take one of two different forms. The first, a **cohort life table**, shows the actual survival of a group of individuals through time. The starting point from which the survival time is measured may be birth, or it may be some other event. For example, a cohort life table may be used to show the mortality experience of an occupational group according to length of employment in the occupation, or the survival pattern of patients following a treatment, such as radiotherapy for small-cell carcinoma of bronchus (Table 16.1). The second type of life table, a **current life table**, is more often used for actuarial purposes and is less common in medical research. This shows the expected survivorship through time of a hypothetical population to which current age-specific death rates have been applied.

The construction of a cohort life table will be described by considering Table 16.1, which shows the survival of patients with small-cell carcinoma of bronchus, month by month following treatment with radiotherapy. This table is based on data collected from a total of 240 patients over a 5-year period. The data themselves are summarized in columns 1–4 of the life table, and the values calculated from them appear in columns 5–8.

Column 1 shows the number of months since treatment with radiotherapy began. Columns 2 and 3 contain the number of patients alive at the beginning of the month and the number who died during the month. For example, 12 of the 240 patients died during the first month of treatment, leaving 228 still alive at the start of the second month.

Table 16.1 Life table showing the survival pattern of 240 patients with small-cell carcinoma of bronchus treated with radiotherapy.

(1) Interval since start of treatment (months)	(2) Number alive at beginning of interval	(3) Deaths during interval	(4) Number lost to follow-up during interval	(5) Number of persons at risk =(2)−(4)/2	(6) Risk of dying during interval =(3)/(5)	(7) Chance of surviving interval =1−(6)	(8) Cumulative chance of survival from start of treatment =(8, previous interval)×(7)
1	240	12	0	240.0	0.0500	0.9500	0.9500
2	228	9	0	228.0	0.0395	0.9605	0.9125
3	219	17	1	218.5	0.0778	0.9222	0.8415
4	201	36	4	199.0	0.1809	0.8191	0.6893
5	161	6	2	160.0	0.0375	0.9625	0.6634
6	153	18	7	149.5	0.1204	0.8796	0.5835
7	128	13	5	125.5	0.1036	0.8964	0.5231
8	110	11	3	108.5	0.1014	0.8986	0.4700
9	96	14	3	94.5	0.1481	0.8519	0.4004
10	79	13	0	79.0	0.1646	0.8354	0.3345
11	66	15	4	64.0	0.2344	0.7656	0.2561
12	47	6	1	46.5	0.1290	0.8710	0.2231
13	40	6	0	40.0	0.1500	0.8500	0.1896
14	34	4	2	33.0	0.1212	0.8788	0.1666
15	28	5	0	28.0	0.1786	0.8214	0.1369
16	23	7	1	22.5	0.3111	0.6889	0.0943
17	15	12	0	15.0	0.8000	0.2000	0.0189
18	3	3	0	3.0	1.0000	0.0000	0.0000

In a study of this kind it is rarely possible to follow all patients until their death. Firstly, some patients may move away from the study area or decide they no longer wish to take part. This is obviously more of a problem the longer the period of follow-up. Secondly, since the entry of patients into the study is usually gradual, those entered towards the end will only have been followed for a short period when the final analysis is made, and unless they have died in this short time they are also lost to follow-up. Thus there will be some patients who are known to have survived up to a certain point in time but whose survivorships past that point are not known. Their survival times are said to be **censored**. Such patients are shown in column 4. The total number of persons at risk of dying during the month, adjusting for these losses, is shown in column 5. This equals the number alive at the beginning of the month minus half the number lost to follow-up, assuming that on average these losses occur half-way through the month.

Column 6 shows the risk of dying during a month, calculated as the number of deaths during the month divided by the number of persons at risk. Column 7 contains the complementary chance of surviving the month, and column 8 the overall, or cumulative, chance of surviving, which equals the chance of surviving up to the end of the previous month multiplied by the chance of surviving the month. For example, the risk of dying during the first month was 12/240 or 0.0500. The chance of surviving was therefore 1 minus this, namely 0.9500. During the second month nine of the remaining 228 patients died, giving a risk of dying of 0.0395 and chance of surviving of 0.9605. This means that patients who had already survived the first month (with a probability of 0.9500) then had a chance of 0.9605 of surviving the second month. The overall chance of surviving two months from the start of treatment was therefore $0.9500 \times 0.9605 = 0.9125$.

Survival curve

In this study all the patients had died by the end of 18 months. Their **survival curve**, drawn using the values in column 8, is shown in Figure 16.1.

Life expectancy

Also of interest is the average length of survival, or **life expectancy**, following the start of treatment. This may be calculated using columns 1 and 8 of the life table. For each interval, the length of the interval is multiplied by the cumulative chance of surviving. The total of these values plus a half gives the life expectancy. (The addition of a half is to allow for the effect of grouping the life table in whole months and is similar to the continuity corrections we

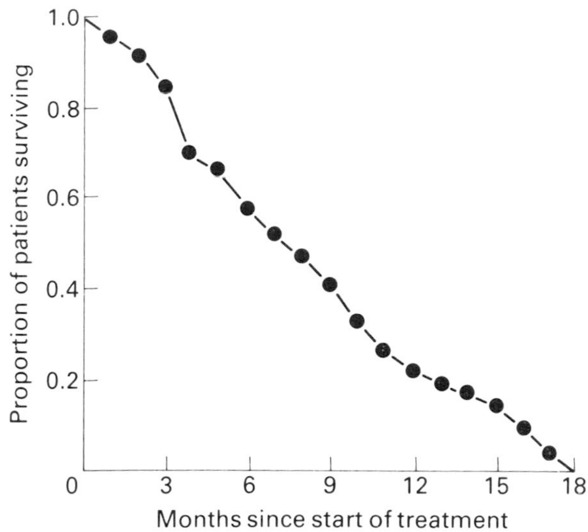

Figure 16.1 Survival curve for patients with small-cell carcinoma of the bronchus treated with radiotherapy. Curve drawn from life table calculations presented in Table 16.1.

have encountered in earlier chapters.)

$$\text{Life expectancy} = \frac{1}{2} + \sum \left(\begin{matrix}\text{number of months}\\ \text{in interval}\end{matrix} \times \begin{matrix}\text{cumulative chance}\\ \text{of survival}\end{matrix} \right)$$

In Table 16.1 all the intervals are of 1 month and so the life expectancy is simply the sum of the values in column 8 plus a half, which equals 7.95 months.

Comparison of life tables

The first step in the comparison of any two life tables is to draw the corresponding survival curves and compare them visually. The statistical significance of any differences observed can then be assessed by the **log rank test**. This is a special application of the Mantel–Haenszel χ^2 procedure, carried out by constructing a separate 2×2 table for each interval of the life tables, in order to compare the proportions dying during each interval. For example, if Table 16.1 showing survival following radiotherapy for small-cell carcinoma of bronchus was compared with a similar life table showing survival following chemotherapy, this procedure would yield 18 2×2 tables, one for each month following treatment. Application of the Mantel–Haenszel

χ^2 test to these tables would summarize the monthly differences between the observed number of deaths following radiotherapy and the expected number, if the survival pattern following radiotherapy were the same as that following chemotherapy. The log rank test can also be extended to adjust for different compositions of the treatment groups, such as different sex ratios or different age distributions. For instance, sex would be taken into account in this example by constructing separate 2×2 tables for males and females for each interval of the life tables, and applying the Mantel–Haenszel χ^2 test to the resulting 36 (2×18) tables. For more details see the papers by Peto *et al.* (1976, 1977), which provide a good practical guide to the analysis of survival data.

An alternative, more sophisticated, approach to the comparison of survival curves is to use **Cox's proportional hazards model**, a method analogous to multiple regression for means and logistic regression for proportions. It is called a proportional hazards model because it assumes that the ratio of the

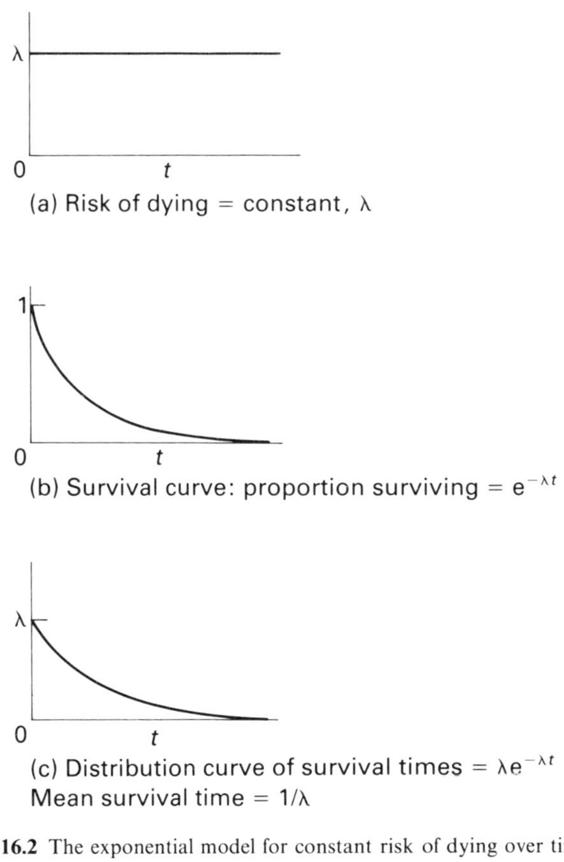

Figure 16.2 The exponential model for constant risk of dying over time (t).

risks of dying in the two groups is constant over time, and that this ratio is the same for different subgroups of the data, such as different age–sex groups. For details see Cox and Oakes (1984).

Patterns of survival

Inspection of column 6 of Table 16.1 shows clearly that the risk of dying from small-cell carcinoma increases with length of time following radiotherapy. Historically much interest has focused on the search for mathematical functions to describe different ways in which the risk of dying (or the **hazard rate**, as it is often called) varies with time. The simplest and best known model is the **exponential**, which asserts a constant risk of death with time. It can be shown mathematically that if a population were subjected to a constant risk of dying, not only would the resulting survival curve be exponential in shape, as illustrated in Figure 16.2, but so would the distribution of survival times, with the life expectancy equalling the reciprocal of the risk of dying. The exponential model is suitable when considering the life of short-lived creatures, such as mosquitos, whose main risk of death is not from ageing but from environmental accidents. It has been used, for example, in developing mathematical models for the transmission of malaria. Other models include the use of the gamma, Weibull, Rayleigh, and Gompertz functions for describing a risk of death that changes with time. Although useful in the mathematical modelling of diseases and survival, these models have not been found to be as helpful in the analysis of survival data as the life table and related methods described above. For more details of the different models, see Cox and Oakes (1984).

CHAPTER 17

The Poisson Distribution

Introduction

We have already met the normal distribution for means and the binomial distribution for proportions. In this chapter we meet the Poisson distribution, named after the French mathematician, which is appropriate for describing the number of occurrences of an event during a period of time, provided that these events occur independently of each other and at random. An example is the number of radioactive emissions detected in a scintillation counter in 5 minutes (*see* Example 17.2). After introducing the Poisson distribution in general, we shall consider its particular application to the analysis of rates, including incidence rates of disease.

The Poisson distribution is also appropriate for the number of particles found in a unit of space, such as the number of malaria parasites seen in a microscope field of a blood slide, provided that the particles are distributed *randomly* and *independently* over the total space. The two properties of randomness and independence must both be fulfilled for the Poisson distribution to hold. For example, the number of *Schistosoma mansoni* eggs in a stool slide will not be Poisson, since the eggs tend to cluster in clumps rather than to be distributed independently.

In Chapter 18 we describe how to assess whether a particular set of data conform with the Poisson distribution, and Example 18.2 presents data which do not comply with the random property. In addition, specific techniques exist to detect disease clustering in time and/or space (see the review by Smith, 1982), such as the possible clustering of cases of childhood leukaemia around nuclear power stations. Such clusters violate what might otherwise be a Poisson distribution.

Definition

The Poisson distribution describes the sampling distribution of the number of occurrences, r, of an event during a period of time (or region of space). It depends upon just one parameter, which is the mean number of occurrences,

μ, in periods of the same length (or in equal regions of space).

$$\text{Probability } (r \text{ occurrences}) = \frac{e^{-\mu}\mu^r}{r!}$$

Most calculators have keys for the three elements of this formula. (e is the mathematical constant 2.71828 . . .). Note that, by definition, both 0! and μ^0 equal 1. The probability of zero occurrences is therefore $e^{-\mu}$.

$$\text{s.e.} = \sqrt{\mu}$$

The standard error for the number of occurrences equals the square root of the mean, which is estimated by the square root of the observed number, $\sqrt{r}$.

Example 17.1

A district health authority which plans to close the smaller of two maternity units is assessing the extra demand this will place on the remaining unit. One factor being considered is the risk that on any given day the demand for admissions will exceed the unit's capacity. At present the larger unit averages 4.2 admissions per day and can cope with a maximum of 10 admissions per day. This results in the unit's capacity being exceeded only on about one day per year. After the closure of the smaller unit the average number of admissions is expected to increase to 6.1 per day. The Poisson distribution can be used to estimate the proportion of days on which the unit's capacity is then likely to be exceeded. For this we need to determine the probability of getting 11 or more admissions on any given day. This is most easily calculated by working out the probabilities of 0, 1, 2 . . . or 10 admissions and subtracting the total of these from 1, as shown in Table 17.1. For example:

$$\text{Probability (three admissions)} = \frac{e^{-6.1}6.1^3}{3!} = 0.0848$$

The calculation shows that the probability of 11 or more admissions in a day is 0.0470. The unit's capacity is therefore likely to be exceeded 4.7% of the time, or about 17 days per year.

Shape

Figure 17.1 shows the shape of the Poisson distribution for various values of

Table 17.1 The probabilities of the number of admissions made during a day in a maternity unit, based on a Poisson distribution with a mean of 6.1 admissions per day.

No. of admissions	Probability
0	0.0022
1	0.0137
2	0.0417
3	0.0848
4	0.1294
5	0.1579
6	0.1605
7	0.1399
8	0.1066
9	0.0723
10	0.0440
Total (0 – 10)	0.9530
11 + (by subtraction)	0.0470

its mean, μ. The distribution is very skewed for small means, when there is a sizeable probability that zero events will be observed. It is symmetrical for large means and is adequately approximated by the normal distribution for values of $\mu = 10$ or more.

Combining counts

Example 17.2

A specimen labelled with a radioactive tracer was counted for 5 minutes in a scintillation counter. The result was 2905 counts. The standard error of this count can be estimated using the Poisson distribution.

$$\text{Count} = 2905$$
$$\text{s.e.} = \sqrt{2905} = 53.9$$

It is more usual to express the result in counts/minute. This gives:

$$\text{Counts/minute} = 2905/5 = 581.0$$
$$\text{s.e.} = 53.9/5 = 10.8$$

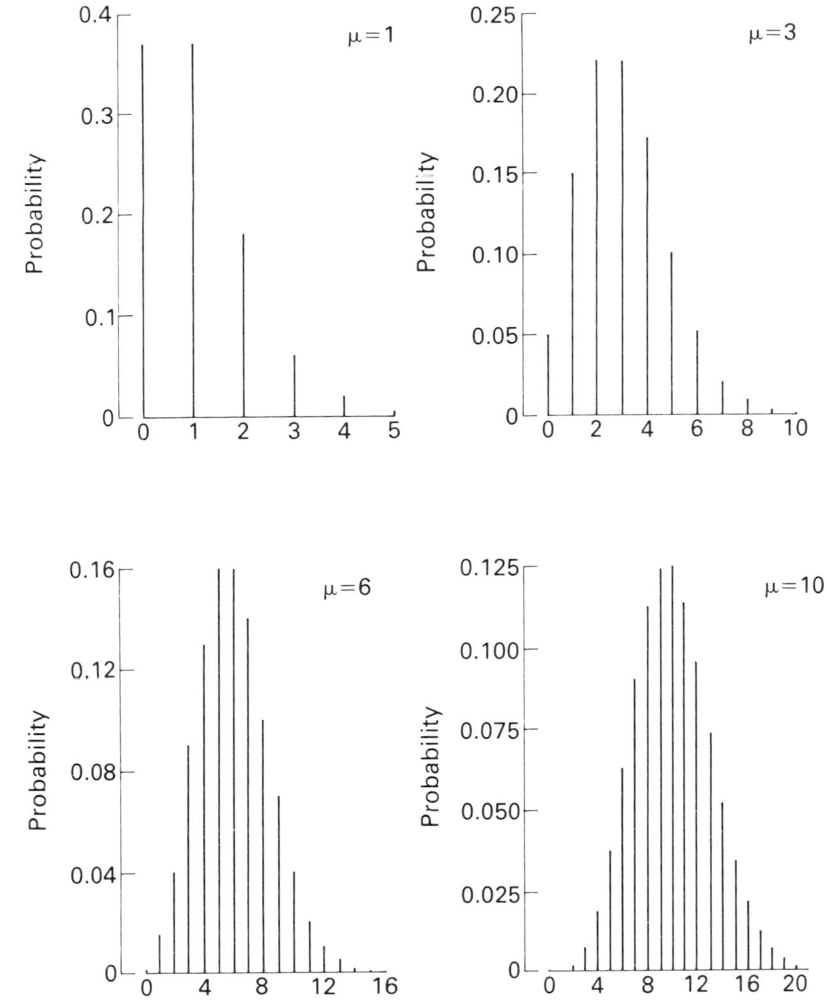

Figure 17.1 Poisson distribution for various values of μ. The horizontal scale in each diagram shows values of r.

A 95% confidence interval for the mean counts per minute may be obtained using the normal approximation, which gives:

$$581.0 \pm 1.96 \times 10.8 = 559.8 \text{ to } 602.2 \text{ counts/minute}$$

Suppose now that three different results were obtained from the scintillation counter based on different time periods, as shown in Table 17.2. The way to combine these results to give an overall value for counts per minute is to *add*

Table 17.2 Results from a scintillation counter.

Result	Count	Time (minutes)
1	1740	3
2	2300	4
3	4055	7
Total	8095	14

the three counts together and divide by the sum of the three time periods.

$$\text{Counts/minute} = 8095/14 = 578.2$$

$$\text{s.e.} = \frac{\sqrt{8095}}{14} = \frac{89.97}{14} = 6.4$$

The mean count/minute is similar to that based on the 5-minute count in Example 17.2. The standard error is smaller, however, as would be expected since the total count was over a longer total time.

The Poisson distribution and rates

In Example 17.2 the variable measured was the *number* of radioactive emissions counted in the scintillation counter during 5 minutes, but we expressed the final result as a *rate* in counts per minute. This was done by dividing both the count and the standard error by 5. We now discuss more generally the use of the Poisson distribution for the analysis of rates, and we introduce another symbol, λ (Greek letter lambda), for the mean rate of occurrence of an event, that is the mean number of occurrences in a *unit* period of time.

$$\text{Mean no. of occurrences per unit time} = \frac{\mu}{t} = \lambda$$

$$\text{s.e.} = \frac{\sqrt{\mu}}{t} = \sqrt{\frac{\lambda}{t}}$$

In Example 17.2, μ is estimated as 2905, t equals 5 and so λ is estimated as 581 counts per minute. Its *standard error* may be calculated either as $\sqrt{\mu}/t$, as was done above, or as $\sqrt{(\lambda/t)}$, which gives:

$$\text{s.e.} = \sqrt{\frac{581}{5}} = 10.8$$

the same as before. The second formula makes clear, however, the way in which the standard error will reduce as the period of observation becomes longer, as λ itself will be the same, on average, for long and short periods.

Analysing incidence rates

An incidence rate is a special type of rate per unit time. Recall from Chapter 15 that it equals the number, r, of new cases of disease in a time period, divided by the total number of person–years at risk (pyar). The Poisson distribution (and its normal approximation) can be used whenever it is reasonable to assume that the cases are occurring independently of each other and randomly in time. This is, of course, less likely to be true for infectious than for non-communicable diseases, but, provided there is no strong evidence of disease clustering, the use is still justified.

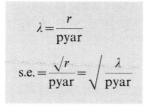

$$\lambda = \frac{r}{\text{pyar}}$$

$$\text{s.e.} = \frac{\sqrt{r}}{\text{pyar}} = \sqrt{\frac{\lambda}{\text{pyar}}}$$

Example 17.3

Fifty-seven lower respiratory infections were recorded during a 2-year morbidity study of children aged less than 5 years in a community in rural Guatemala. Five hundred children were initially enrolled in the study, but because of migration, new births, passing the age of 5, and losses to follow-up, the number under surveillance varied with time. The total child–years of follow-up was 873. The incidence rate of lower respiratory infection, expres-

Table 17.3 Incidence of lower respiratory infection among children aged less than 5 years, according to their housing conditions.

Housing condition	No. of infections	Child–years at risk	Incidence rate/ 1000 child–years
Poor	33	355	93.0
Good	24	518	46.3
Overall	57	873	65.3

sed per 1000 child–years at risk, was estimated to be:

$$\lambda = 57/873 \times 1000 = 65.3 \text{ per 1000 child–years}$$

with

$$\text{s.e.} = \frac{\sqrt{57}}{873} \times 1000 = 8.6$$

The 95% confidence interval equals:

$$65.3 \pm 1.96 \times 8.6 = 48.4 \text{ to } 82.2 \text{ infections per 1000 child–years}$$

Comparison of two incidence rates

A normal test can be used to compare two incidence rates, $\lambda_1 = r_1/\text{pyar}_1$ and $\lambda_2 = r_2/\text{pyar}_2$. The formula with a *continuity correction* is:

$$z = \frac{|\lambda_1 - \lambda_2| - [1/(2\text{pyar}_1) + 1(2\text{pyar}_2)]}{\sqrt{[\lambda(1/\text{pyar}_1 + 1/\text{pyar}_2)]}}, \quad \lambda = \frac{r_1 + r_2}{\text{pyar}_1 + \text{pyar}_2}$$

where λ is the overall incidence rate in the two groups and $|\lambda_1 - \lambda_2|$ means the *size* of the difference ignoring its sign.

Example 17.4

The children analysed in Example 17.3 were subdivided into two groups, those living in 'good' housing and those living in 'poor' housing. The results were as shown in Table 17.3. The incidence rate of lower respiratory infections was considerably higher among children with poor living conditions than among those with good living conditions; 93.0 and 46.3 per 1000 child–years, respectively. Since the rates are expressed per *thousand* child–years, the pyar elements in the formula must also be expressed in units of 1000. This gives:

$$z = \frac{|93.0 - 46.3| - (1/1.036 + 1/0.710)}{\sqrt{[65.3 \times (1/0.518 + 1/0.355)]}} = 2.52$$

The difference is highly significant ($P \simeq 0.01$).

CHAPTER 18

Goodness of Fit of Frequency Distributions

Introduction

We have met several theoretical distributions. In this chapter we discuss how to assess whether the distribution of an observed set of data agrees with a particular theoretical model. For example, do the data conform with the normal distribution, a requirement of many statistical methods. We consider this first. The second part of the chapter is more general. It describes the chi-squared goodness of fit test for testing the significance of the differences between an observed frequency distribution and the distribution predicted by a theoretical model.

Goodness of fit to a normal distribution

An assumption of normality underlies many statistical methods. This can be checked by comparing the shape of the observed frequency distribution with that of the normal distribution. Formal significance testing is rarely necessary, as in general we are only interested in detecting marked departures from normality; most methods are robust against moderate departures. If the sample size is large, visual assessment of the frequency distribution is often adequate. For example, the shape of the histogram in Figure 18.1(a) seems reasonably similar to that of the normal distribution, while that in Figure 18.1(b) is clearly positively skewed.

A graphical technique, which can be used for samples of any size, is the **probit plot**. This is a scatter diagram comparing the percentage points of the observed frequency distribution with the corresponding points (called probits) of the standard normal distribution. The probit plot is linear if the data are normally distributed and curved if they are not.

For example, Table 18.1 gives the frequency distribution of the haemoglobin measurements made on 70 women, illustrated in Figure 18.1(a). None of the women had a haemoglobin level below 8 g/100 ml. Only one, that is 1.4% of the total, had a level below 9 g/100 ml. The value of the standard normal distribution corresponding to this percentage can be found from Table A6. It equals -2.20, which is said to be the **probit** of 1.4%. Many people add 5 to the value obtained to ensure that the probit is always

Table 18.1 Frequency distribution of haemoglobin levels of 70 women. Also shown is the cumulative distribution with corresponding probits.

Haemoglobin (g/100 ml)	No. of women	Cumulative number	Cumulative (%)	Probit
<8	0	0	0.0	—
8–	1	1	1.4	−2.20
9–	3	4	5.7	−1.58
10–	14	18	25.7	−0.65
11–	19	37	52.9	0.07
12–	14	51	72.9	0.61
13–	13	64	91.4	1.37
14–	5	69	98.6	2.20
15–	1	70	100.0	—
16+	0			

positive, but this is not necessary and will not be done here.

Probit = Value of standard normal distribution corresponding to cumulative percentage (+5, optional)

Three women had a haemoglobin level between 9 and 10 g/100 ml making a total of four (5.7%) with levels below 10 g/100 ml. Using Table A6 again, the probit corresponding to 10 g/100 ml is found to be −1.58. Similarly 18 women (25.7%) had haemoglobin levels below 11 g/100 ml. Numbers accumulated in this way are called **cumulative**. The cumulative values of the rest of the frequency distribution are shown in Table 18.1, together with their corresponding probits. Recommendations differ on what probit values should be used for 0% and 100%, none of which is entirely satisfactory. Very little information is lost by simply omitting them as done here.

Figure 18.1(c) shows the probits plotted against haemoglobin levels. Note that, for example, the probit −2.20 is plotted against 9 g/100 ml (and not 8 g/100 ml) since it corresponds to the percentage of the distribution *below* 9 g/100 ml. The plot is linear, confirming the visual impression that the data are normally distributed. In contrast, Figure 18.1(d) shows the non-linear probit plot corresponding to the positively skewed distribution of triceps skinfold measurements shown in Figure 18.1(b).

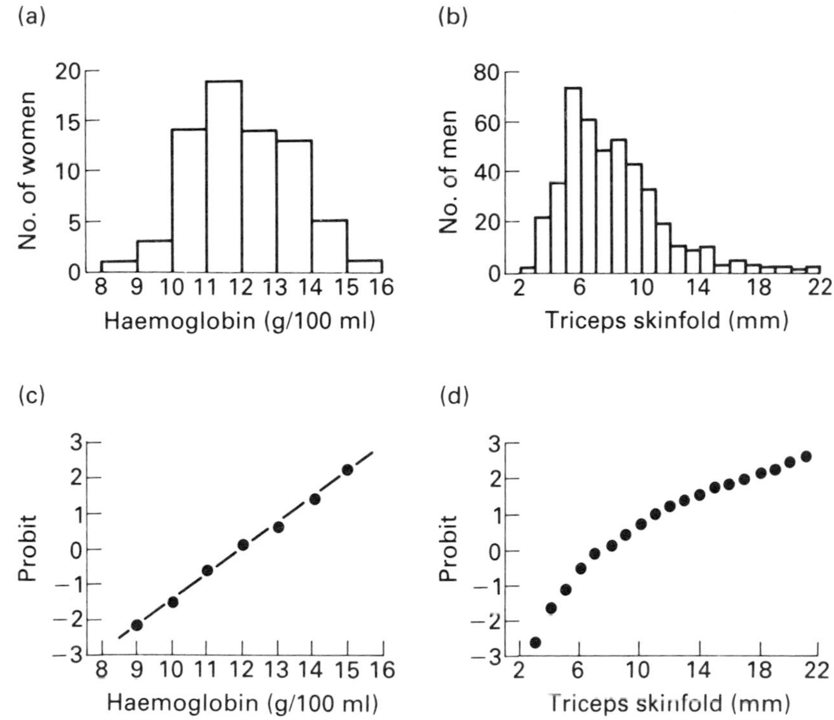

Figure 18.1 Frequency distributions with probit plots to assess the normality of the data. (a) and (c) Haemoglobin levels of 70 women. Normally distributed. Probit plot linear. (b) and (d) Triceps skinfold measurements of 440 men. Positively skewed. Probit plot non-linear.

The probit plot can also be drawn using individual observations rather than a frequency distribution. This is particularly useful for small samples. The observations are arranged in ascending order. Their associated cumulative percentages are:

$$100 \times 1/n,\ 100 \times 2/n,\ 100 \times 3/n,\ \ldots\ 100 \times n/n$$

where n is the sample size. For example, if there were 24 observations, the cumulative percentages would be 4.2%, 8.4%, 13.2% . . . 100%. The corresponding probits are found as above, and are plotted against the individual values.

Chi-squared goodness of fit test

It is sometimes useful to test whether an observed frequency distribution differs significantly from a postulated theoretical one, such as the Poisson distribution. This may be done by comparing the observed and expected frequencies using a chi-squared test. The form of the test is exactly the same as that for contingency tables, that is:

$$\chi^2 = \sum \frac{(O-E)^2}{E}$$

but the calculation of the *degrees of freedom* is different. These equal the number of groups in the frequency distribution minus 1, minus the number of parameters estimated from the data. For example, if an exponential distribution is fitted to survival times, then just one parameter is estimated, namely λ, the reciprocal of the mean survival. In fitting a normal distribution, two parameters are needed, its mean, μ, and its standard deviation, σ. In some cases no parameters are estimated from the data, either because the theoretical model requires no parameters, as in Example 18.1, or because the parameters are specified as part of the model.

$$\text{d.f.} = \begin{array}{l}\text{number of groups}\\ \text{in frequency}\\ \text{distribution}\end{array} - \begin{array}{l}\text{number of}\\ \text{parameters}\\ \text{estimated}\end{array} - 1$$

Calculation of expected numbers

The first step in carrying out a chi-squared goodness of fit test is to estimate the parameters needed for the theoretical distribution from the data. The next step is to calculate the expected numbers in each category of the frequency distribution, by multiplying the total frequency by the probability that an individual value falls within the category.

$$\begin{array}{c}\text{Expected}\\ \text{frequency}\end{array} = \begin{array}{c}\text{total}\\ \text{frequency}\end{array} \times \begin{array}{c}\text{probability individual}\\ \text{falls within category}\end{array}$$

For discrete data, the probability is calculated by a straightforward application of the distributional formula, as illustrated for the Poisson distribution in Example 18.2. For continuous data, it is calculated from the cumulative distribution. For example, if the data are survival times of mosquitos, then the probability that an individual mosquito dies during its third day of life equals the probability that it survives to the start of the second day minus the probability that it survives to the start of the third day.

Validity

The chi-squared goodness of fit test should not be used if more than a small proportion of the *expected* frequencies are less than 5 or if any are less than 2. This can be avoided by combining adjacent groups in the distribution.

Example 18.1

Table 18.2 examines the distribution of the final digit of the weights recorded in a survey, as a check on their accuracy. Ninety-six adults were weighed and their weights recorded to the nearest tenth of a kilogram. If there were no biases in recording, such as a tendency to record only whole or half kilograms, one would expect an equal number of 0s, 1s, 2s . . . and 9s for the final digit, that is 9.6 of each. The agreement of the observed distribution with this can be tested using the chi-squared goodness of fit test. There are 10 frequencies and no parameters have been estimated.

$$\chi^2 = \sum \frac{(O-E)^2}{E} = 9.84, \quad \text{d.f.} = 10 - 0 - 1 = 9$$

9.84 is between the 25% and 50% points for the χ^2 distribution with 9 degrees of freedom. The observed frequencies therefore agree well with the theoretical ones, suggesting no recording bias.

Table 18.2 Check on the accuracy in a survey of recording weight.

Final digit of weight	Observed frequency	Expected frequency	$\frac{(O-E)^2}{E}$
0	13	9.6	1.20
1	8	9.6	0.27
2	10	9.6	0.02
3	9	9.6	0.04
4	10	9.6	0.02
5	14	9.6	2.02
6	5	9.6	2.20
7	12	9.6	0.60
8	11	9.6	0.20
9	4	9.6	3.27
Total	96	96.0	9.84

Example 18.2
It is thought that multiple invasion of erythrocytes is more likely to occur with *Plasmodium falciparum* than with the other malaria parasites. Table 18.3 shows data collected to ascertain whether these parasites attack certain red blood cells preferentially, or whether multiple infections are simply chance events. Fifty thousand erythrocytes were examined in the blood film of a patient with *falciparum* malaria, and the number of parasites in each recorded.

Table 18.3 The observed frequency distribution of the number of parasites per erythrocyte in the blood film of a patient with *Plasmodium falciparum* malaria, compared with a Poisson distribution of the same mean. With permission from Wang (1970) *Transactions of the Royal Society of Tropical Medicine and Hygiene* **64**, 268–70.

No. of parasites per erythrocyte	Observed distribution	Poisson distribution	$\frac{(O-E)^2}{E}$
0	40 000	39 726.7	1.9
1	8621	9137.1	29.2
2	1259	1050.8	41.3
3	99	80.6	4.2
4	21	4.6	58.5
5+	0	0.2	0.2
Total	50 000	50 000.0	135.3

If the infection of individual red blood cells is a chance event, the distribution of number of parasites per cell would be Poisson. This hypothesis can be tested using the chi-squared goodness of fit test. The first step is to calculate, μ, the mean number of parasites per erythrocyte. This equals:

$$\frac{0\times 40\,000+1\times 8621+2\times 1259+3\times 99+4\times 21}{50\,000}=\frac{11\,520}{50\,000}=0.23$$

The next is to calculate the expected numbers of erythrocytes with 0, 1, 2, 3, 4 or 5+ parasites using a Poisson distribution with this mean. The results are shown in Table 18.3. For example, the probability that a cell has two parasites is:

$$\frac{e^{-\mu}\mu^2}{2!}=\frac{e^{-0.23}0.23^2}{2!}=0.021015$$

The expected number of cells out of the total of 50 000 with two parasites is therefore:

$$50\,000 \times 0.021015 = 1050.8$$

Finally the observed and expected frequencies are compared. It can be seen from Table 18.3 that there are many fewer cells than expected with just one or two parasites and many more with three or four parasites, suggesting that the parasites attack cells preferentially rather than at random. The chi-squared value is highly significant.

$$\chi^2 = 135.3, \quad \text{d.f.} = 6 - 1 - 1 = 4, \quad P < 0.001$$

CHAPTER 19

Transformations

Introduction

The assumptions underlying a statistical method may not always be satisfied by a particular set of data. For example, a distribution may be positively skewed rather than normal, the standard deviations of two groups may be very different contraindicating the use of the *t* test in comparing their means, or the relationship between two variables may be curved rather than linear. We will now describe how such problems can often be overcome simply by transforming the data to a different scale of measurement. By far the most common choice is the logarithmic transformation, which will be described in detail. A summary of the use of other transformations will be presented at the end of the chapter.

Logarithmic transformation

When a logarithmic transformation is applied to a variable, each individual value is replaced by its logarithm.

$$u = \log x$$

where x is the original value and u the transformed value. This can only be used with positive values, since logarithms of negative numbers do not exist, and the logarithm of zero is minus infinity. There are sometimes instances, however, when a logarithmic transformation is indicated, as in the case of parasite counts, but the data contain some zeros as well as positive numbers. This problem is solved by adding 1 to each value before transforming. (Note that 1 must then also be subtracted after the final results have been converted back to the original scale.)

The logarithmic transformation has the effect of stretching out the lower part of the original scale, and compressing the upper part, as shown in Figure 19.1. For example, on a logarithmic scale, the distance between 1 and 10 is the same as that between 10 and 100 and as that between 100 and 1000; they are all 10-fold differences.

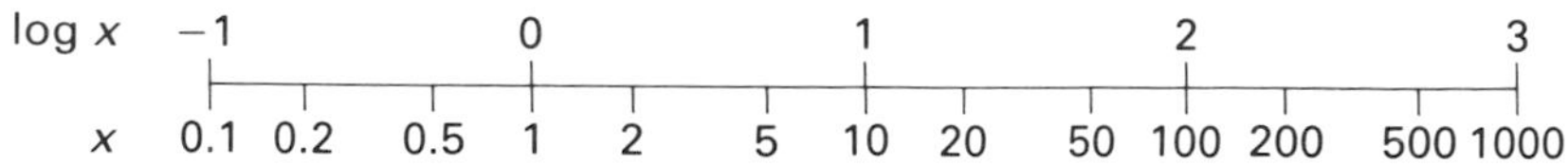

Figure 19.1 The logarithmic transformation.

Positively skewed distributions

The logarithmic transformation will therefore tend to normalize positively skewed distributions, as illustrated by Figure 19.2, which is the result of applying a logarithmic transformation to the triceps skinfold data presented in Figure 18.1(b). The histogram is now symmetrical and the probit plot linear, showing that the transformation has removed the skewness and normalized the data. Triceps skinfold is said to have a **lognormal distribution**.

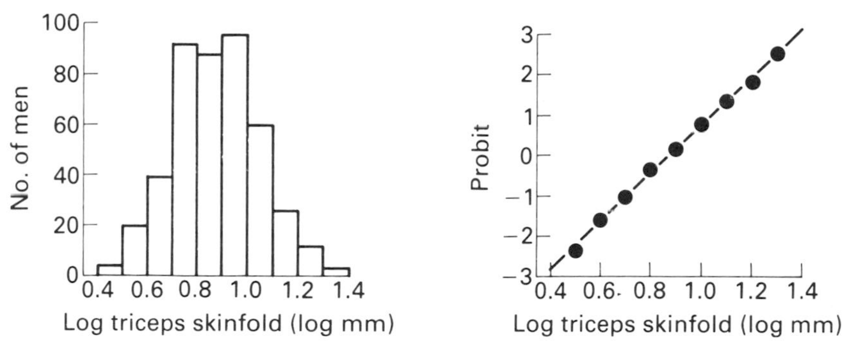

Figure 19.2 Lognormal distribution of triceps skinfold measurements of 440 men. Compare with Figure 18.1.

Unequal standard deviations

The mechanics of using a logarithmic transformation will be described by considering the data of Table 19.1(a), which show a higher mean urinary β-thromboglobulin (β-TG) excretion in 12 diabetic patients than in 12 normal subjects. These means cannot be compared using a t test since the standard deviations of the two groups are very different. The right-hand columns of the table show the observations after a logarithmic transformation. For example, log(4.1)=0.61. Logarithms to any base may be used; the effect will be the same. The usual choice is to use base 10, as done here, or base e, that is natural logarithms (ln).

The transformation has had the effects both of equalizing the standard deviations (they are 0.26 and 0.28 on the logarithmic scale) and of removing skewness in each group (*see* Figure 19.3). The t test may now be used, showing

Table 19.1 Comparison of urinary β-thromboglobulin (β-TG) excretion in 12 normal subjects and in 12 diabetic patients. Adapted from results by van Oost *et al.* (1983) *Thrombosis and Haemostasis* **49**, 18–20, with permission.

(a) Original and logged data

	β-TG (ng/day/100 ml creatinine)		Log β-TG (log ng/day/100 ml creatinine)	
	Normals	Diabetics	Normals	Diabetics
	4.1	11.5	0.61	1.06
	6.3	12.1	0.80	1.08
	7.8	16.1	0.89	1.21
	8.5	17.8	0.93	1.25
	8.9	24.0	0.95	1.38
	10.4	28.8	1.02	1.46
	11.5	33.9	1.06	1.53
	12.0	40.7	1.08	1.61
	13.8	51.3	1.14	1.71
	17.6	56.2	1.25	1.75
	24.3	61.7	1.39	1.79
	37.2	69.2	1.57	1.84
Mean	13.5	35.3	1.06	1.47
s.d.	9.2	20.3	0.26	0.28
n	12	12	12	12

(b) Calculation of t test on logged data

$$s=\sqrt{[(11\times 0.26^2+11\times 0.28^2)/22]}=0.27$$

$$t=\frac{1.06-1.47}{0.27\sqrt{(1/12+1/12)}}=-3.72,\quad \text{d.f.}=22,\quad P\simeq 0.001$$

(c) Results reported in original scale.

	Geometric mean β-TG	95% c.i.	Geometric s.d.
Normals	11.5	7.8, 17.0	1.8
Diabetics	29.5	19.5, 44.7	1.9

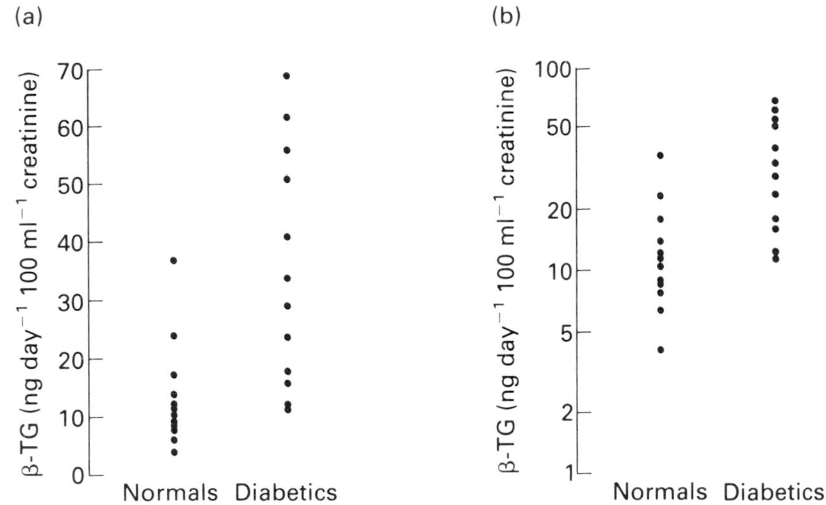

Figure 19.3 β-Thromboglobulin data (Table 19.1) drawn using (a) a linear scale and (b) a logarithmic scale. Note that the logarithmic scale has been labelled in the original units.

that mean log β-TG is significantly higher for the diabetic patients. The details of the calculations are presented in Table 19.1(b).

Geometric mean and confidence interval

When using a transformation, *all analyses* are carried out on the transformed values, u. It is important to note that this includes the calculation of any confidence intervals. For example, the mean log β-TG of the normals was 1.06 log ng/day/100 ml. Its 95% confidence interval equals:

$$1.06 \pm 2.20 \times 0.26/\sqrt{12} = 0.89 \text{ to } 1.23 \text{ ng/day/100 ml}$$

(Note that 2.20 is the 5% point of the t distribution with 11 degrees of freedom.)

When reporting the final results, however, it is sometimes clearer to transform them back into the original units by taking antilogs, as done in Table 19.1(c). The antilog of the mean of the transformed values is called the **geometric mean**.

$$\text{Geometric mean (GM)} = \text{antilog}\,(\bar{u}) = 10^{\bar{u}}$$

For example, the geometric mean β-GT of the normal subjects is:

$$\text{Antilog}(1.06) = 10^{1.06} = 11.5 \text{ ng/day/100 ml}$$

The geometric mean is always smaller than the corresponding arithmetic mean (unless all the observations have the same value, in which case the two measures are equal). Unlike the arithmetic mean, it is not overly influenced by the very large values in a skewed distribution, and so gives a much better representation of the average in this situation.

Its confidence interval is calculated by antilogging the confidence limits calculated on the log scale. For the normal subjects, the 95% confidence interval for the geometric mean therefore equals:

$$\text{antilog}(0.89),\quad \text{antilog}(1.23) = 10^{0.89}, 10^{1.23}$$
$$= 7.8, 17.0 \text{ ng/day/100 ml}$$

Note that the confidence interval is not symmetric about the geometric mean. Instead the ratio of the upper limit to the geometric mean, $17.0/11.5 = 1.5$, is the same as the ratio of the geometric mean to the lower limit, $11.5/7.8 = 1.5$. This reflects the fact that a standard deviation on a log scale corresponds to a multiplicative rather than an additive error on the original scale.

For the same reason, the antilog of the standard deviation is not readily interpretable, and is therefore not commonly used. There are some situations, however, such as in large tables summarizing several different variables, when because of its conciseness, the antilog of the standard deviation may be preferred to the confidence interval. The term **geometric standard deviation** has been suggested (Kirkwood 1979).

Non-linear relationship

Figure 19.4(a) shows how the frequency of 6-thioguanine (6TG) resistant lymphocytes increases with age. The relationship curves upwards and there is greater scatter of the points at older ages. Figure 19.4(b) shows how using a log transformation for the frequency has both linearized the relationship and stabilized the variation.

In this example, the relationship curved upwards and the y variable (frequency) was transformed. The equivalent procedure for a relationship which curves downwards is to take the logarithm of the x value.

Analysis of titres

Many serological tests, such as the haemagglutination test for rubella antibody, are based on a series of doubling dilutions, and the strength of the most dilute solution that provides a reaction is recorded. The results are called **titres**, and are expressed in terms of the strengths of the dilutions $\frac{1}{2}, \frac{1}{4}, \frac{1}{8}, \frac{1}{16}, \frac{1}{32}$, etc. For convenience, we will use the terminology more loosely, and refer

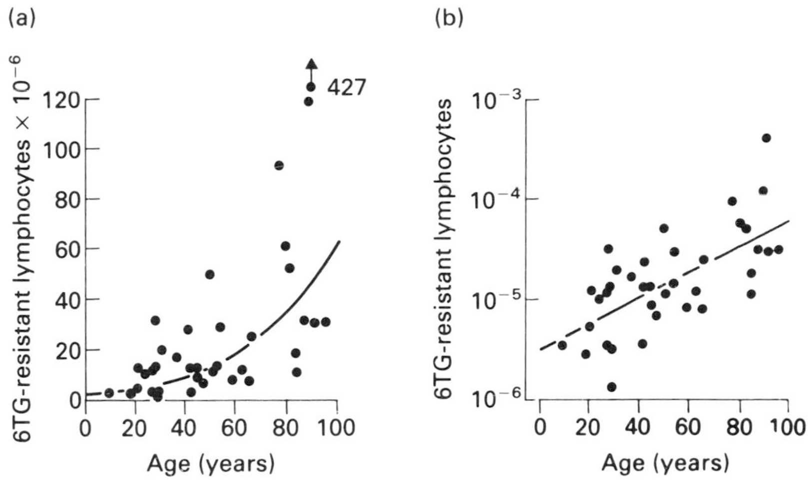

Figure 19.4 Relationship between frequency of 6TG-resistant lymphocytes and age for 37 individuals drawn using (a) a linear scale and (b) a logarithmic scale for frequency. With permission from Morley *et al.* (1982) *Mechanisms of Ageing and Development* **19**, 21–6.

instead to the reciprocals of these numbers, namely 2, 4, 8, 16, 32, etc., as titres. Titres tend to be positively skewed, and are therefore best analysed using a logarithmic transformation. This is accomplished most easily by replacing the titres by their corresponding dilution numbers. Thus titre 2 is replaced by dilution number 1, titre 4 by 2, titre 8 by 3, titre 16 by 4, titre 32 by 5, and so on. This is equivalent to taking logarithms to the base 2 since, for example, $8=2^3$ and $16=2^4$.

$$u = \text{dilution number} = \log_2 \text{titre}$$

All analyses are carried out using the dilution numbers. The results are then transformed back into the original units by calculating 2 to the corresponding power.

For example, Table 19.2 shows the measles antibody levels of 10 children one month after vaccination for measles. The results are expressed as titres with their corresponding dilution numbers. The mean dilution number is $\bar{u}=4.4$. We antilog this by calculating $2^{4.4}=21.1$. The result is the **geometric mean titre** and equals 21.1.

$$\text{Geometric mean titre} = 2^{\text{mean dilution number}}$$

Table 19.2 Measles antibody levels one month after vaccination.

Child no.	Antibody titre	Dilution no.
1	8	3
2	16	4
3	16	4
4	32	5
5	8	3
6	128	7
7	16	4
8	32	5
9	32	5
10	16	4

Choice of a transformation

As previously mentioned, the logarithmic transformation is by far the most frequently applied. It is appropriate for removing positive skewness and is used on a great variety of variables including incubation periods, survival times, parasite counts, titres, dose levels, concentrations of substances, and ratios. There are, however, alternative transformations for skewed data as summarized in Table 19.3. For example, the **reciprocal transformation** is stronger than the logarithmic, and would be appropriate if the distribution were considerably more positively skewed than lognormal, while the **square root transformation** is weaker. Negative skewness, on the other hand, can be removed by using a **power transformation**, such as a square or a cubic transformation, the strength increasing with the order of the power.

There is a similar choice of transformation for making standard deviations more similar, depending on how much the size of the standard error increases with increasing mean. (It rarely decreases.) Thus, the logarithmic transformation is appropriate if the standard deviation increases approximately in proportion to the mean, while the reciprocal is appropriate if the increase is steeper, and the square root if it is less steep.

Table 19.3 also summarizes the different sorts of simple non-linear relationships that might occur. The choice of transformation depends on the shape of the curve and whether the y variable or the x variable is to be transformed.

Table 19.3 Summary of different choices of transformations. Those removing positive skewness are called group A transformations, and those removing negative skewness group B.

Situation	Transformation	
Positively skewed distribution (group A)		
Lognormal	Logarithmic ($u = \log x$)	
More skewed than lognormal	Reciprocal ($u = 1/x$)	
Less skewed than lognormal	Square root ($u = \sqrt{x}$)	
Negatively skewed distribution (group B)		
Moderately skewed	Square ($u = x^2$)	
More skewed	Cubic ($u = x^3$)	
Unequal variation		
s.d. proportional to mean	Logarithmic ($u = \log x$)	
s.d. proportional to mean^2	Reciprocal ($u = 1/x$)	
s.d. proportional to $\sqrt{\text{mean}}$	Square root ($u = \sqrt{x}$)	
Non-linear relationship	y variable and/or	x variable
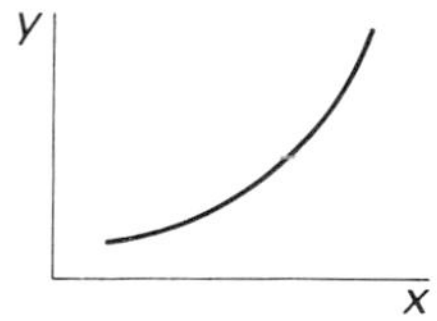	Group A	Group B
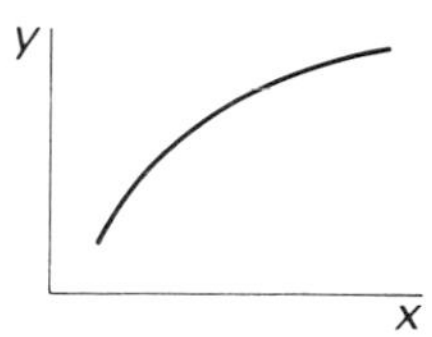	Group B	Group A
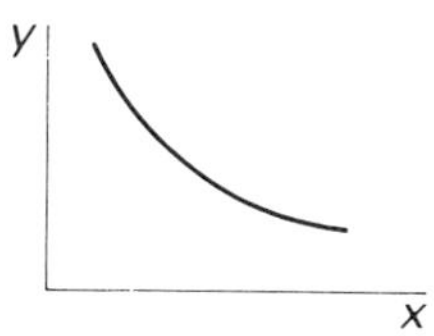	Group A	Group A
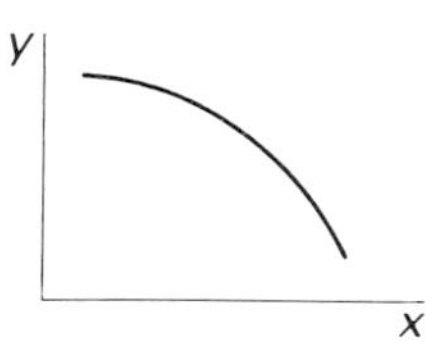	Group B	Group B

Finally, we will briefly mention two transformations which relate specifically to proportions. These are the logistic (or logit) transformation introduced in Chapter 14 and the probit transformation described in Chapter 18. The main effect of both transformations is to convert the restricted range of the proportion scale, that is from zero to 1, to an infinite scale.

CHAPTER 20

Non-parametric Methods

Introduction

Non-parametric methods are an alternative set of statistical techniques for analysing numerical data that make no assumptions about the underlying distribution, for example the normality of the data. They are particularly useful when there is obvious non-normality in a small data set which cannot be corrected by a suitable transformation.

Many non-parametric methods were originally developed as quick and easy methods but it was discovered that their performance compared remarkably well with that of the traditional parametric methods such as t tests. They are almost as efficient in detecting genuine differences when the parametric assumptions are satisfied and considerably more so when they are not. As will be seen, non-parametric methods are indeed very easy to use provided the data consist of no more than about 50 cases. With the widespread use of calculators and computers, however, this is less of an advantage than it once was. They have two main disadvantages. Firstly, their primary concern is significance testing and, although it is possible to derive confidence intervals using them, the procedures are complicated and tedious to perform. Secondly, they are less easily extendable to the more complex situations. For these reasons the emphasis in this book is on the use of parametric methods when these are valid.

The main non-parametric methods are listed in Table 20.1 together with their parametric counterparts. The three most common ones, the Wilcoxon signed rank test, the Wilcoxon rank sum test and Spearman's rank correlation, will be described using examples previously analysed by the more traditional techniques. For the other non-parametric methods the reader is referred to Siegel (1956). Strictly speaking the χ^2 methods described in Chapters 13 and 14 are also non-parametric, but as they are the standard methods for the analysis of proportions and contingency tables they are generally included among the traditional methods.

Wilcoxon signed rank test

This is the non-parametric equivalent of the paired t test. It uses the signs and relative magnitudes of the data but not their actual values. For example,

Table 20.1 Summary of the main non-parametric methods.

Non-parametric method	Use	Parametric equivalent
Sign test	Simplified form of Wilcoxon signed rank test	
Wilcoxon signed rank test	Test of difference between paired observations	Paired t test
Wilcoxon rank sum test	Comparison of two groups	Two-sample t test
Mann–Whitney U test	Alternatives to the Wilcoxon rank sum test which give identical results	Two-sample t test
Kendall's S test		Two-sample t test
Kruskal–Wallis one-way analysis of variance	Comparison of several groups	One-way analysis of variance
Friedman two-way analysis of variance	Comparison of groups, defined by their values on two variables	Two-way analysis of variance
Spearman's rank correlation	Measure of association between two variables	Correlation coefficient
Kendall's rank correlation	Alternative to Spearman's rank correlation	Correlation coefficient
χ^2 goodness of fit test	Comparison of an observed frequency distribution with a theoretical one (*see* Chapter 18)	
Kolmogorov–Smirnov tests		
One-sample	Alternative to χ^2 goodness of fit test	
Two-sample	Comparison of two frequency distributions	

consider the results in Table 20.2, which shows the number of hours of sleep obtained by 10 patients with a sleeping drug and with a placebo, and the differences between them. The Wilcoxon signed rank test consists of four basic steps.

1 Exclude any differences which are zero. Put the remaining differences in ascending order of magnitude, ignoring their signs and give them **ranks** 1, 2, 3, etc. If any differences are equal, as is the case for patients 1 and 2, average their ranks. The ranks are also shown in Table 20.2.

2 Count up the ranks of the positive differences and of the negative differences and denote these sums by T_+ and T_- respectively.

$$T_+ = 3.5 + 10 + 7 + 5 + 8 + 6 + 2 + 9 = 50.5$$
$$T_- = 3.5 + 1 = 4.5$$

3 If there were no difference in effectiveness between the sleeping drug and the placebo then the sums T_+ and T_- would be similar. If there were a

Table 20.2 Results of a placebo-controlled clinical trial to test the effectiveness of a sleeping drug (same data as in Table 6.1), with ranks for use in the Wilcoxon signed rank test.

Patient	Hours of sleep		Difference	Rank (ignoring sign)
	Drug	Placebo		
1	6.1	5.2	0.9	3.5*
2	7.0	7.9	−0.9	3.5*
3	8.2	3.9	4.3	10
4	7.6	4.7	2.9	7
5	6.5	5.3	1.2	5
6	8.4	5.4	3.0	8
7	6.9	4.2	2.7	6
8	6.7	6.1	0.6	2
9	7.4	3.8	3.6	9
10	5.8	6.3	−0.5	1

* Tied 3rd and 4th and so ranks averaged.

difference then one sum would be much smaller and one sum would be much larger than expected. Denote the smaller sum by T.

$$T = \text{smaller of } T_+ \text{ and } T_-$$

In this example, $T = 4.5$.

4 The Wilcoxon signed rank test is based on assessing whether T, the smaller of the observed sums, T_+ and T_-, is smaller than could be expected by chance. Compare the value obtained with the critical values for the 5%, 2% and 1% significance levels given in Table A7. Note that the appropriate sample size, N, is the number of differences that were ranked rather than the total number of differences, and does not therefore include the zero differences.

$$N = \text{number of non-zero differences}$$

In contrast to the usual situation, a result is significant if it is *smaller* than the critical value shown. In this example, the sample size is 10 and the 5%, 2%, and 1% percentage points are 8, 5, and 3 respectively. The result is therefore significant at the 2% level, since 4.5 is smaller than 5, indicating that the sleeping drug was more effective than the placebo.

Wilcoxon rank sum test

This is one of the non-parametric equivalents of the *t* test. Its use will be described by considering the data in Table 20.3, which shows the birth weights of children born to 15 non-smokers and 14 heavy smokers. The Wilcoxon rank sum test consists of three basic steps.

1 Rank the observations from both groups together in ascending order of magnitude, as shown in the table. If any of the values are equal, average their ranks.

2 Add up the ranks in the group with the smaller sample size. In this case it is the heavy smokers, and their ranks sum to 163. If the two groups are of the same size either one may be picked.

T = sum of ranks in group with smaller sample size

Table 20.3 Comparison of birth weights of children born to 15 non-smokers with those of children born to 14 heavy smokers (same data as in Table 7.1), with ranks for use in the Wilcoxon rank sum test.

Non-smokers ($n=15$)		Heavy smokers ($n=14$)	
Birth weight (kg)	Rank	Birth weight (kg)	Rank
3.99	27	3.18	7
3.79	24	2.84	5
3.60*	18	2.90	6
3.73	22	3.27	11
3.21	8	3.85	26
3.60*	18	3.52	14
4.08	28	3.23	9
3.61	20	2.76	4
3.83	25	3.60*	18
3.31	12	3.75	23
4.13	29	3.59	16
3.26	10	3.63	21
3.54	15	2.38	2
3.51	13	2.34	1
2.71	3		
	Sum = 272		Sum = 163

* Tied 17th, 18th, and 19th and so ranks averaged.

3 Compare this sum with the critical ranges given in Table A8, which is arranged somewhat differently to the tables for the other significance tests. Look up the row corresponding to the sample sizes of the two groups, in this case row 14, 15. The range shown for the 5% significance level is 164 to 256 and corresponds to *non-significant values*. In other words, sums of 164 and below or 256 and above are significant at the 5% level. The sum of 163 in this example is just below the lower limit of 164 which means that the birth weights of the children born to the heavy smokers are significantly lower than those of the children born to the non-smokers ($P < 0.05$).

Spearman's rank correlation

This is a non-parametric measure of the degree of association between two numerical variables. The parametric equivalent is the correlation coefficient, sometimes known as **Pearson's product moment correlation**, described in Chapter 9. The values of each variable are independently ranked and the measure is based on the differences between the pairs of ranks of the two variables. This will be illustrated using the data in Table 20.4 on the relationship between plasma volume and body weight in eight healthy men. There are four basic steps.

1 Rank the values of each of the variables separately, as shown in the table. If any of the values are equal, average their ranks. If there is a high proportion

Table 20.4 Relationship between plasma volume and body weight in eight healthy men (same data as in Table 9.1), with ranks and their differences for use in calculating the Spearman rank correlation.

	Body weight		Plasma volume		Difference between	Squared difference
Subject	Value (kg)	Rank	Value (litre)	Rank	ranks d	d^2
1	58.0	1	2.75	2	−1	1
2	70.0	5	2.86	4	1	1
3	74.0	8	3.37	7	1	1
4	63.5	3	2.76	3	0	0
5	62.0	2	2.62	1	1	1
6	70.5	6	3.49	8	−2	4
7	71.0	7	3.05	5	2	4
8	66.0	4	3.12	6	−2	4
						$\Sigma d^2 = 16$

of tied values, an adjusted formula is needed for calculating the correlation. The reader is referred to Siegel (1956) for details.

2 Calculate the differences, d, between each pair of ranks, square them and add them up. In this example the sum Σd^2 equals 16.

3 Calculate Spearman's rank correlation which is denoted by r_s.

$$r_s = 1 - \frac{6\Sigma d^2}{n(n^2-1)}$$

where n is the number of subjects. This correlation will have a value between -1 and 1, and its interpretation is similar to that of the ordinary correlation coefficient. 1 corresponds to perfect agreement between the ranks of the two variables, zero corresponds to no relationship, and -1 corresponds to a perfect inverse agreement between the ranks.

In this example:

$$r_s = 1 - \frac{6 \times 16}{8 \times (8^2 - 1)} = 0.81$$

4 The significance of the association is tested by comparing r_s with the critical values given in Table A9. The value of 0.81 based on eight pairs is significant at the 5% level, since 0.81 is larger than the critical value of 0.738, confirming a positive association between plasma volume and body weight.

Alternatively, *when there are 10 or more pairs*, the significance may be assessed using a t test in the same way as described for the ordinary correlation coefficient.

$$t = r_s \sqrt{\left[\frac{n-2}{1-r_s^2}\right]}, \quad \text{d.f.} = n-2$$

CHAPTER 21

Planning and Conducting an Investigation

Introduction

The emphasis so far has been on how to analyse data once they have been collected. In the remaining seven chapters of the book we discuss how to plan and conduct an investigation. Adequate consideration of the issues involved is of paramount importance, since no amount of sophisticated analysis can salvage either a poorly designed or a badly carried out study. This chapter gives an overview of the design issues involved, and Chapter 22 discusses potential sources of error that can arise. Chapters 23–25 then consider the different types of study design in more detail, and Chapter 26 addresses the issue of sample size, that is how to calculate the number of individuals that need to be studied in order to answer the questions of interest. Finally, Chapter 27 contains an introduction to the use of computers.

It is impossible in a limited amount of space to cover all aspects in detail. The aim has been to include sufficient description that the reader will become familiar with the concepts involved and be able both to design simple studies and to assess the adequacy of the study designs of investigations reported in the literature. For more in-depth discussions the specialist books listed in the bibliography, for example on clinical trials and case–control studies, should be consulted.

Finally, it should be noted that there is no universal agreement on how to classify different types of study objectives and designs, nor are there always clear-cut boundaries between different subcategories. I have chosen to adopt a scheme which I believe affords a convenient, practical way of assessing what is an appropriate design(s) for a particular situation, rather than to focus on the historical perspective of the evolution of different designs.

Objectives of study

The starting point of any investigation must be to define clearly its objectives, since these will determine the appropriate study design and the type of data needed. Objectives may be categorized into one of three main types as listed below. An investigation usually has several objectives, which can of course be of different types.

1 **Estimation** of certain features of a population. For example, what percentage of children have received a full course of vaccination by their third birthday, or what is the average number of diarrhoeal episodes per year experienced by under-5-year-olds in Bangladesh?
2 Investigation of the **association** between a factor of interest and a particular outcome, such as disease or death. For example, are breast-fed infants less likely to die than non breast-fed infants, or are respiratory infections more common among children whose parents smoke?
3 **Evaluation** of a drug or therapy or of an intervention aimed at reducing the incidence (or severity) of disease. For example, does the administration of BCG reduce the risk of recurrence of bladder warts, or does the use of sleeping nets reduce the risk of malaria, and if so does spraying the nets with insecticide afford additional protection?

Analysis of vital statistics

Occasionally it is possible to answer objectives using vital statistics or other routinely collected health statistics. Of historical interest, the first recorded analysis of vital statistics was carried out by John Graunt of London, who published his *Natural and Political Observations upon the Bills of Mortality* in 1662. Graunt demonstrated, among other things, the excess of males over females in both births and deaths, the high infant mortality rates, and the seasonal variation in mortality. In 1693, Edmund Halley used these same Bills of Mortality to construct the first life table (*see* Chapter 16). Graunt was ahead of his time, however, and the tradition of such analyses was not established until the middle of the nineteenth century when William Farr became the first Registrar General of England and Wales. Farr applied vital statistics data to many problems of public health, including the comparison of mortality rates between various occupational groups.

Examination of routinely collected vital statistics data on births, deaths, and morbidity may also provide the first clue to an association between a disease and its cause. For example, the increase in mortality from lung cancer and its possible association with the increased frequency of cigarette smoking was initially noted from vital statistics data. This hypothesis was subsequently tested with specially designed case–control and cohort studies (*see below*).

Observational studies

In general, it will be necessary to carry out a special study to collect the relevant data to answer the specific objectives. Estimation and association objectives lead to studies which are **observational** in nature; the natural history of disease is observed with no attempt made in the study to alter it. Evaluation objectives may be answered by either observational or **experimental** studies, depending on the type of measure being evaluated and whether it is already in use. An example of the former would be the assessment of the efficacy of BCG vaccination against tuberculosis in an area with an active immunization programme where BCG is routinely administered, since the choice of who received or did not receive vaccination would not be under the investigator's control. In contrast, the trial of a new malaria vaccine would probably be experimental.

Observational study designs may be divided into three major groups, cross-sectional, longitudinal (including cohort) and case–control studies. The sampling schemes appropriate for cross-sectional and longitudinal studies are described in detail in Chapter 23. In general the aim should be to use a method which gives every person an equal chance of being selected, that is to use an **equal probability scheme**. People may be selected individually or in clusters, although a larger total sample size is required for the latter. The available resources and logistic difficulties often mean, however, that it is not possible to examine a sufficient number of clusters to gain a representative picture, and results are not uncommonly based on a survey in just one community. Judgement of representativeness is then subjective rather than statistical. This is less of a problem if the main objective is to investigate associations than if it is to obtain estimates. Methods of measuring association are described in Chapter 24, which also considers design issues specific to case–control studies.

Cross-sectional study

A **cross-sectional** study is carried out at just one point in time or over a short period of time. Cross-sectional studies are relatively quick, cheap and easy to carry out, and straightforward to analyse. Since they provide estimates of the features of a community at just one point in time, however, they are suitable for measuring prevalence but not incidence of disease, and associations found may be difficult to interpret. For example, a survey on onchocerciasis showed that blind persons were of lower nutritional status than non-blind. There are two possible explanations for this association. The first is that those of poor nutritional status have lower resistance and are therefore more likely to become blind from onchocerciasis. The second is that poor nutritional status is a consequence rather than a cause of the blindness, since blind persons are not as able to provide for themselves. Longitudinal data are necessary to decide which is the better explanation.

Longitudinal study

In a **longitudinal** study individuals are followed over time, which makes it possible to measure incidence of disease and changes over time and easier to study the natural history of disease. In some situations it is possible to obtain follow-up data on births, deaths, and episodes of disease by **continuous monitoring**, for example by monitoring registry records in populations where registration of deaths is complete. Occasionally the acquisition of data may be **restrospective**, being carried out from past records. More commonly it is **prospective** and, for this reason, longitudinal studies have often been alternatively termed prospective studies.

In the majority of cases, the simplest way to carry out a longitudinal study is to conduct **repeated cross-sectional surveys** at fixed intervals and to enquire about, or measure, changes that have taken place between surveys, such as births, deaths, migrations, changes in weight or antibody levels, or the occurrence of new episodes of disease. The interval chosen will depend on the factors being studied. For example, to measure the incidence of diarrhoea, which is characterized by repeated short episodes, data may need to be collected weekly to ensure reliable recall. To monitor child growth, on the other hand, would require only monthly or 3-monthly measurements.

The population under study may be either dynamic or fixed. In a **dynamic** situation, individuals leave the study when they no longer conform to the population definition, while new individuals satisfying the conditions may join. An example would be the study of incidence of diarrhoea in under-5-year-olds, in which monitoring of children would cease when they attained their fifth birthday, while newborns would be recruited into the population as they were born. In a **fixed** situation, on the other hand, the population is defined at the onset and, apart from deaths, migrations, and other losses to follow-up, its composition remains unchanged throughout the study. A fixed population is often called a **cohort**, such as the **birth cohort** of 1984, that is all people born in 1984. Another example would be the industrial cohort of all people employed in the nuclear power industry between 1970 and 1974.

Set against the many benefits of the longitudinal design are several disadvantages. Firstly, the analysis is more complicated than that of a cross-sectional one and may require sophisticated data processing facilities. The linkage of results between surveys is not a trivial task, and allowance must be made for migrations, deaths, and new entrants. Adjustment may also be necessary for the ageing of the study group over time. Secondly, the longer the study period and the more surveys that are carried out, the higher the drop-out and non-response rate and the greater the problem of incomplete data. Finally, longitudinal studies tend to be more costly and to pose many logistic problems in their execution.

Case–control study

A **case–control** study is used to investigate the association between a certain factor and a particular disease. The design is very different to other types of studies because the sampling is carried out according to disease status rather than exposure status. A group of individuals identified as having the disease, the **cases**, is compared with a group not having the disease, the **controls**. For example, in assessing whether breast-feeding mediates against infant death, cases would comprise children who died during the first year of life, and controls might be children living in the same area and of the same age and sex as the cases. If the hypothesis were true, it would be found that the cases were less likely to have been breast-fed than the controls.

Case–control studies are particularly appropriate for uncommon diseases, for which they require a considerably smaller sample size than the corresponding cross-sectional or longitudinal studies. They are relatively cheap, quick and easy to carry out, and lead to a measure of relative incidence of disease (*see* Chapter 24) among those exposed and non-exposed to the factor of interest. The complexities of the method lie instead in the careful consideration needed in the design in order to minimize the types of bias that may occur, namely selection, misclassification, and recall bias, and in the relatively sophisticated analysis required. In particular the choice of appropriate controls is often a controversial issue. Case–control studies are therefore most successful at detecting large effects, since it is easier to be convinced that these are real rather than artefacts of the design. Finally, case–control studies (like cross-sectional studies) are not suitable if the disease itself affects the risk factor of interest as well as possibly being a consequence of it, as in the case of poor nutritional status as a risk factor for diarrhoea.

Experimental studies

Medical investigations that are experimental in nature may be categorized into three main groups according to the nature of the measure being evaluated.

1 **Clinical trials** of drugs or other therapeutic measures.

2 **Vaccine trials.**

3 **Intervention trials** of:

(a) Prophylactic regimes (other than vaccines), for example giving antimalarials during the first 5 years of life to children in an area endemic for malaria. Such studies are sometimes called **prophylactic trials**.

(b) Preventive measures, such as the use of sleeping nets as a protection against malaria.

Their design is discussed in detail in Chapter 25. The essential ingredient is that the allocation of individuals to the different experimental groups is under the investigator's control, and that this allocation should be such as to ensure that the groups are as similar as possible in all respects other than the regime/ measure being evaluated. The use of a **double-blind controlled trial** (*see* Chapter 25) is recommended in order to avoid bias.

Questionnaire design

In most studies it will be necessary to prepare a specially designed record form or questionnaire for collecting the data. This should be kept as brief as possible, and the temptation to ask every conceivable question should be resisted. Overlong questionnaires are tiring for interviewer and interviewee alike, and may lead to unreliable responses. Questions should be clear and unambiguous and written exactly as they are to be read out. Technical jargon or long words should be avoided, as should negative questions, leading questions, and hypothetical questions.

Careful thought should be given to the order in which information is collected and to whether the questionnaire should be self-administered or completed by an interviewer. There should be a logical progression through the form which is easily followed. Questions are best arranged in sections. It should be clearly indicated whenever the completion of a section is dependent on the response to a previous question, and the starting point of the next section should be easily identifiable. It is best to minimize the number of skips or jumps which can occur, since too many can be confusing, and sections can be accidentally missed. The questionnaire should be clearly labelled with the title of the study and with the respondent's name and study identification number. These should be repeated on the top of each page. The next section usually consists of general identifying information such as age, sex, and address. In general it is a good idea to arrange subsequent sections in order of importance of the information to the study, so that the most important information is collected when the interviewer and interviewee are freshest and least bored. Any sensitive questions are, however, probably best left to the end.

Open and closed questions

Questions may be in one of two forms, open or closed. **Open questions** are used to search for information, and the interviewer records the replies in a freely written form. There are no preconceived ideas about what the possible responses might be. In a **closed question**, on the other hand, the response is restricted to one of a specified list of possible answers. This list should include a category for 'Other' with space to write in the details and a category for 'Don't know'. The interviewer may either lead the respondent through the list category by category, or ask the question in an open form and then tick the category which most closely corresponds to the answer given. Open and closed forms each have advantages and disadvantages, and the choice very much depends on the particular context. Responses to closed questions are considerably more straightforward to process, but open questions can yield more detailed and in-depth information. One possibility is to use an open form during the pilot phase of the study and to use the results of this to draw up the list of answers for a closed question form for the main study.

Coding

Numerical data should be recorded in as much detail as possible and as individual values rather than precoded on the questionnaire into groups. Consider the example of age. The preferred option is to record date of birth and later to calculate age from this and the date of interview. The next best is to record the respondent's age in, for example, years for adults, months for young children, weeks for infants, and days for newborns. The least satisfactory approach is simply recording in which age-group, such as 0–4, 5–9, 10–14, 15–24, 25–44, 45–64 or 65+ years, the respondent belongs. The units of any measurements should also be clearly specified, for example whether weight is to be recorded in kilograms or pounds, and the number of digits of accuracy required should also be indicated. With closed questions, the corresponding numerical codes should be printed alongside the listed choice of responses. With open questions, it will be necessary to code the replies after the questionnaire has been completed and space should be allowed for this.

If data are to be entered onto a computer then this should be borne in mind when designing the questionnaire. For example, it may speed up the data entry procedure if all the information to be entered is coded into boxes arranged down the right-hand side of the form. In most cases it will be necessary to assign numerical codes to the responses to non-numerical variables, such as code 1 for male and 2 for female. One box is needed for each digit (or letter), the total number of boxes required for a variable being determined by the number of digits in the maximum response likely to be recorded for the variable. Where possible the use of code zero should be avoided, since on many computer systems and in many statistical software packages it is impossible to distinguish zero from a blank response, meaning no data.

Multiple response questions

Multiple response questions require special consideration. They can be dealt with in two different ways. For example, in rural West Africa a family may use one or more of eight possible sources (rainwater, borehole, well, spring, river, lake, pond, stream) for their drinking water. The first method is to assign a separate coding box to each possible response, in this case eight. Each box would contain either code '1' for source used or '2' for source not used. Thus if a family used rainwater and also collected water from a river, the rainwater box (number 1) and the river box (number 5) would contain code 1, while the other six boxes would contain code 2. The second method is to instead assign codes 1 to 8 to the eight different sources and to decide on the maximum number of responses any family is likely to give. Suppose we decided that three responses was the limit. We would then allocate three separate coding boxes to the question and enter in these the code numbers of the sources named. The family using rainwater and river water would be coded as 1 (rainwater) in box 1 and as 5 (river) in box 2. Box 3 would be left blank. The codes should be entered either in numerical order, as done here, or in some other logical order, such as amount of usage of source.

Data checking

Each questionnaire should be carefully checked after completion, and again once the data have been entered onto the computer. The importance of this should not be overlooked. Checking should take place as soon after data collection as possible in order to allow the maximum chance of any resulting queries being resolved. Checks are basically of two sorts, range checks and consistency checks. **Range checks** exclude, for example, the erroneous occurrence of code 3 for sex, which should only be code 1 (male) or 2 (female). **Consistency checks** detect impossible combinations of data such as a pregnant man, or a 3-year-old weighing 70 kg. Scatter diagrams showing the relationship between two variables are particularly helpful in doing this, as they allow odd combinations of, for example, height and weight to be easily spotted.

Three basic precautions are recommended to minimize errors occurring during the handling of data. The first is to avoid any unnecessary copying of data from one form to another. The second is to use a **verification** procedure during data entry. Data are entered twice, preferably by two different persons, as this gives an independent assessment of any poorly written figures. The two data sets are then compared and any discrepancies resolved. The third is to check all calculations carefully, either by repeating them or, for example, by checking that subtotals add to the correct overall total. When using a computer, all procedures should be tried out initially on a small subset of the data and the results validated by hand.

CHAPTER 22

Sources of Error

Introduction

It is important to be aware of the various ways errors may creep into the design, conduct, and analysis of a study in order to be able to take steps to minimize their occurrence. We will start by distinguishing between the two main types, **systematic** and **random**. For example, consider the results of an experiment to assess the agreement between different nurses in taking blood pressure measurements. Four nurses each measured the same 10 volunteers. Inspection of the results showed that although nurses A, B, and C did not always obtain the same individual values, there was no obvious pattern to the disagreements and their average results were similar. Thus any errors occurring were *random* ones. In contrast, nurse D's readings were consistently lower than those of her colleagues, and her average result was 10 mmHg lower. She was committing a *systematic* error and her average estimate was incorrect, being lower than it should have been. Her result is said to be **biased**.

Every stage of an investigation is susceptible to systematic errors. These are potentially serious, since the bias they cause may lead to invalid conclusions being drawn. Random errors, on the other hand, give rise to reduced precision, but not in general to invalidity. They occur during data collection through questionnaire or equipment faults, observer error, and responder mistakes, and during data processing through coding, copying, data entry, programming, and calculating errors. Errors also arise through inappropriate choice of methods of analysis and incorrect interpretation of the results.

Bias may be classified into three main categories: selection bias, confounding bias, and information bias. These are all more likely to occur in observational studies than in experimental ones, where they can be avoided by the use of a randomized controlled double-blind design (*see* Chapter 25). They are particularly a problem in case–control designs. We will now briefly consider each type of bias. For a more detailed discussion consult Kleinbaum *et al.* (1982). We will then define the two parameters, sensitivity and specificity, which are used to assess the ability of a procedure to correctly classify an individual's appropriate disease (or exposure) status. Finally, we will consider the special problem of bias arising from a phenomenon called regression to the mean.

Selection bias

Selection bias may result from one (or both) of two different design inadequacies in the way subjects are selected for study. The first is if subjects selected for study differ in some systematic way from those not selected. The main causes are a high non-response rate, loss to follow-up, or an inappropriate choice of sampling frame. For example, in many countries a study of severe diarrhoea based on hospitalized cases would exclude particularly acute cases who died before reaching hospital, and would selectively exclude those living far from the hospital, and families of lower socioeconomic or educational status, since these tend to be poorer users of health facilities. The second type is selection bias in a comparative study resulting from an inappropriate choice of comparison groups, differential medical surveillance or hospitalization, leading to a higher likelihood of being diagnosed as a case in the exposed compared to the non-exposed groups (**Berkson's fallacy**), differential survival, or differential follow-up.

Confounding bias

Confounding bias occurs whenever there are important differences between the groups being compared that are also related to the variable of interest. An example has already been discussed in Chapter 14 in Table 14.4 where we wished to compare the prevalence of leptospirosis among adults from rural and urban areas. In this case sex was a confounding variable, since not only were the prevalence rates considerably higher for males than for females, but the sex compositions of the rural and urban samples were very different. We overcame this problem by constructing separate 2×2 tables for males and females and using the Mantel–Haenszel χ^2 test.

Confounding is a potential problem in all studies. It can be controlled for in the design using the techniques of matching described in Chapters 24 and 25, and in experimental studies by randomization of individuals to the different experimental groups. Unlike all other types of bias it can also be corrected for in the analysis.

Information bias

Information bias results from systematically incorrect measurements or responses or from differential misclassification of disease or exposure status of participants. It has a variety of causes. These include questionnaire faults, observer errors, respondent errors, and instrumental errors. Questionnaire faults may result from culturally inappropriate questions, ambiguous wording, or too many questions. Observer errors may be due to misunderstanding of procedures, misinterpretation of responses, or simply mistakes. More seriously, observer errors may bias the findings of a study as a result of differences in assessment, in probing or in the interpretation of doubtful answers if the exposure or disease status of the respondent is known to the observer. This is particularly likely if the interviewer is also aware of the hypothesis under study.

Respondent errors may arise through misunderstanding, faulty recall, giving the perceived 'correct' answer, or through lack of interest. In some instances the respondent may deliberately give the wrong answer because, for example, of embarrassment in questions connected with sexually transmitted diseases or because of suspicion that answers would be passed to income tax authorities. Finally, examples of instrumental errors are faulty calibration, contaminated reagents, incorrect dilution or mixing of reagents, or an inaccurate diagnostic test.

Sensitivity and specificity

The ability of a procedure to classify individuals correctly into one of two categories, such as diseased or non-diseased, exposed or non-exposed, positive or negative, at high risk or not, is assessed by two parameters, sensitivity and specificity. **Sensitivity** is the proportion of true *positives* that are correctly identified as such and is 1 minus the **false negative rate**. **Specificity** is the proportion of true *negatives* that are correctly identified as such and is 1 minus the **false positive rate**. For example, Table 22.1 shows the results of a pilot study to assess parents' ability to recall the correct BCG immunization status of their children, as compared to health authority records. Of the 60 children who had in fact received BCG immunization, almost all, 55, were correctly identified as such by their parents, giving a sensitivity of 55/60 or 91.7%. In contrast 15 of the 40 children with no record of BCG immunization

Table 22.1 Comparison of parents' recall of the BCG immunization status of their children with that recorded in the health authority records.

BCG immunization according to health authority records	BCG immunization according to parents		
	Yes	No	Total
Yes	55	5	60
No	15	25	40
Total	70	30	100

were claimed by their parents to have been immunized, giving a specificity of 25/40 or 62.5%.

The measures of sensitivity and specificity are particularly important in assessing **screening tests**. Note that there is an inverse relationship between the two measures, tightening (or relaxing) criteria to improve one will have the effect of decreasing the magnitude of the other. Where to draw the line between them will depend on the nature of the study. For example, in designing a study to test a new leprosy vaccine, it would be important initially to exclude any lepromatous patients. One would therefore want a test with a high success rate of detecting positives, or in other words a highly sensitive test. One would be less concerned about specificity, since it would not matter if a true negative was incorrectly identified as positive and so excluded. In contrast, for the detection of cases during the post-vaccine (or placebo) follow-up period, one would want a test with high specificity, since it would then be more important to be confident that any positives detected were real, and less important if some were missed.

Regression to the mean

Regression to the mean refers to a phenomenon first observed by Galton when he noticed that the heights of sons tended to be closer to the overall mean than the heights of their fathers. Thus, tall fathers tended to have sons shorter than themselves, while the opposite was true for short fathers. Failure to appreciate this phenomenon can lead to misleading interpretation of findings in two circumstances. The first is if the difference between two repeated measurements is related to the first measurement. The second is if only individuals in the extreme of a distribution are selected for treatment and follow-up. These will be explained by considering the repeated measurement of blood pressure and the assessment of antihypertensive drugs in reducing blood pressure.

Figure 22.1 shows the relationship between two diastolic blood pressure readings taken 6 months apart on 50 volunteers. It can be seen that apart from random variation there is good agreement between the two readings. However, when the difference between the two readings is related to the initial reading, a different picture is observed (Figure 22.2). It appears that there is a downward gradient, and that those with a high initial level have a reduced blood pressure 6 months later while the opposite is true for those with an initial low level. This is a spurious finding. It is entirely caused by the fact that there is a mathematical relationship between the difference ($BP_2 - BP_1$) and the initial reading BP_1, BP_1 contributing to both variables.

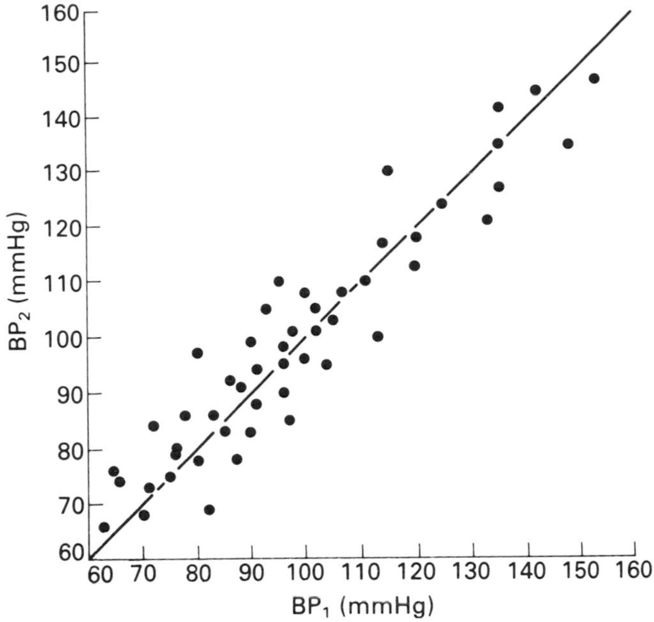

Figure 22.1 The relationship between two diastolic blood pressure readings taken six months apart on 50 volunteers, showing little change on average. The straight line is the relationship that would be seen if the readings on the two occasions were the same.

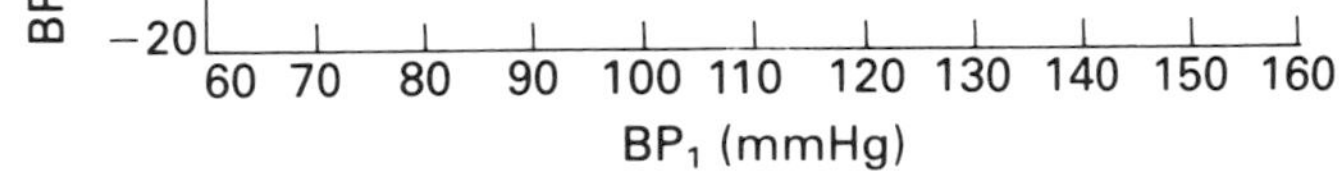

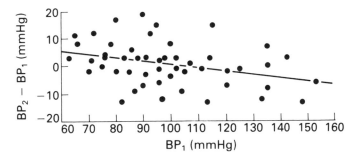

Figure 22.2 Change in diastolic blood pressure plotted against initial value. An artificial negative correlation ($r = -0.35$, d.f. $= 48$, $P < 0.02$) is observed. The straight line is the regression line corresponding to this association.

Yet one does sometimes want to be able to assess whether, for example, a treatment-induced change is related to the initial value. Let us consider the implications of regression to the mean for clinical trials of antihypertensive drugs. Such trials are usually confined to people with initial high blood pressure, say above 120 mmHg. It can be seen from Figure 22.2 that if such people were followed for a period of time and remeasured their blood pressures would on average have decreased, even in the absence of any treatment. Thus it is essential to have a control group of persons with initially similar levels of blood pressure and to assess any apparent reduction in mean blood pressure of the treated group by a comparison with the mean reduction observed in the control group.

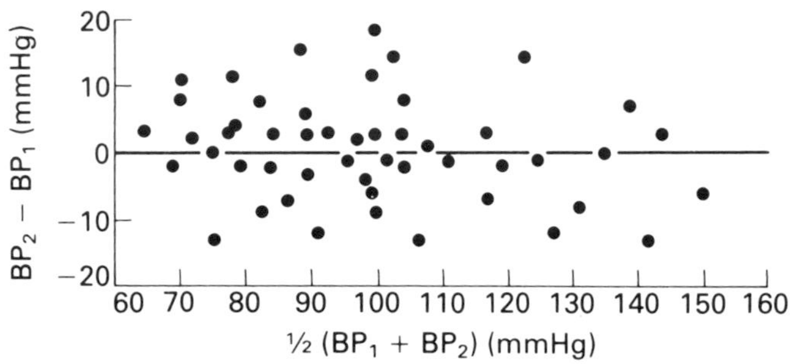

Figure 22.3 Change in diastolic blood pressure plotted against the average of the initial and final readings. The correlation is not significant ($r = -0.19$, d.f. $= 48$, $P \simeq 0.2$), showing the true picture of no relationship between $BP_2 - BP_1$ and blood pressure level.

To assess whether the drug's effect is related to the blood pressure level, an approach suggested by Oldham (1962) may be used. The difference ($BP_2 - BP_1$) is plotted against the *average* of the initial and final blood pressure readings $\frac{1}{2}(BP_1 + BP_2)$ rather than against the initial reading. A negative correlation of these variables would imply a tendency for people with high blood pressure to show a larger decrease than those with low blood pressure, while a positive correlation would imply the opposite. Figure 22.3 shows a plot of ($BP_2 - BP_1$) against $\frac{1}{2}(BP_1 + BP_2)$ for the data in Figure 22.1. The correlation is not significant, confirming that Oldham's method has overcome the spurious apparent association between blood pressure reduction and initial blood pressure which was caused by regression to the mean.

CHAPTER 23

Sampling Methods

Introduction

The role of cross-sectional and longitudinal surveys was outlined in Chapter 21. We will now describe the different sampling schemes that may be employed. Occasionally a complete **census** of the population is carried out, but more often only a **sample** is investigated. The main reasons for this are economy of time and money. The disadvantages are that an estimate based on a sample will be subject to sampling error, as discussed in Chapters 1 and 3, and may be biased if the sample is not representative of the population. The choice of the size of sample to study so that the error is within specified limits is described in Chapter 26. Random selection of the sample is recommended to avoid any selection bias, conscious or otherwise, and the appropriate methods will now be briefly outlined. Randomization alone will not, however, overcome other potential sources of bias, as described in Chapter 22. For example, non-response of some of the selected individuals may cause bias, as non-responders may well differ from responders with respect to the aspects under study.

Simple random sampling

In simple random sampling, the first step is to draw up a list of all the individuals in a population and to number them. This list is called the **sampling frame**. Next the required number of individuals is selected; each has the same chance of being chosen. This could be achieved by labelling a card for each individual, shuffling them, and then selecting the appropriate number of cards. A more convenient method is to use a **table of random numbers** such as Table A10. First look at the total number in the population and see how many digits it comprises. Random numbers with this number of digits are then selected. For example, if the population consists of 2432 members, four-digit numbers are needed. Finally an *arbitrary* starting point in the table is chosen (it is bad practice always to start in the same place) and numbers are read off, moving down columns or across rows as preferred, until the required number of *different* individuals have been chosen. If a selected number is larger than the population total, or if it is zero, it is simply ignored. Note that the arrangement of numbers in pairs in the table is for presentation purposes only. Alternatively, computer-generated random numbers may be used. The use of the random number facility available on many calculators is, however, not recommended, as these have often been found not to yield a truly random distribution.

Example 23.1
Consider the selection of a sample of 10 houses from a village of 268 houses. Table 23.1 shows an extract of random numbers from Table A10 to illustrate how this is done. As the total number of houses is 268, three-digit numbers are required. These are formed by using a pair of numbers followed by the first digit of the adjacent pair. Starting at the top left-hand corner and reading down columns, the first number is 173. The next number, 770, is too large and is ignored. The next number in the required range is 074 or 74. This is continued until 10 different numbers are chosen. These are underlined in the table. Thus the houses to be studied are numbers 5, 74, 79, 83, 138, 166, 173, 201, 242, and 259.

Table 23.1 Extract of random tables from Table A10, illustrating the choice of 10 numbers between 1 and 268.

17	37	93	23	78	87	35	20	96	43
77	04	74	47	67	21	76	33	50	25
98	10	50	71	75	12	86	73	58	07
52	42	*07	44	38	15	51	00	13	42
49	17	46	09	62	90	52	84	77	27
79	83	86	19	62	06	76	50	03	10
83	11	46	32	24	20	14	85	88	45
07	45	32	14	08	32	98	94	07	72
00	56	76	31	38	80	22	02	53	53
42	34	07	96	88	54	42	06	87	98
13	89	51	03	74	17	76	37	13	04
97	12	25	93	47	70	33	24	03	54
16	64	36	16	00	04	43	18	66	79
45	59	34	68	49	12	72	07	34	45
20	15	37	00	49	52	85	66	60	44

* 074 has already been selected.

Systematic sampling

For convenience, selection from the sampling frame is sometimes carried out systematically rather than randomly, by taking individuals at regular intervals down the list, the starting point being chosen at random. For example, to select a 5%, or 1 in 20, sample of the population, the starting point is chosen randomly from numbers 1 to 20, and then every 20th person on the list is taken. Suppose 13 is the random number selected, then the sample would comprise individuals 13, 33, 53, 73, 93, etc.

A systematic sample will be equivalent to a random one provided that there is no underlying pattern in the order of individuals on the list. Random sampling is preferred, however, as no assumptions are necessary about the structure of the population.

More complex sampling schemes

There are many situations in which a simple random sample is not appropriate and a more complex sampling scheme is necessary. Such situations arise when (i) a sampling frame does not already exist and it would be too costly or impracticable to compile one, (ii) the population is spread over a wide area and the travel costs and time involved in covering the whole area are prohibitive, and (iii) the population consists of quite distinct subgroups.

The three basic types of more complex sampling schemes are **stratified, multi-stage** and **cluster** sampling. These may be used alone or in combination and will now be described. In general the aim should be to apply these schemes in such a way as to give every individual an equal chance of being selected, that is to use them with an **equal probability selection method, epsem** for short.

An important point to appreciate is that the population value is estimated directly by the overall sample value only for an epsem scheme. If a non-equal probability method is used, the method of estimating the population value will be different (*see* Example 23.2). In both instances, the calculation of the standard error will depend on the particular sampling scheme used. For a full discussion of the practical issues involved, the reader is referred to Lutz (1986) and to Moser and Kalton (1971) and for the theoretical details to Cochran (1977) and to Stuart (1984).

Stratified sampling

Stratified sampling is used when the population consists of distinct subgroups, or **strata**, which differ with respect to the feature under study and which are themselves of interest. Commonly occurring examples are different age–sex groups or different regions of a country. A simple random sample is taken from each stratum to ensure that they are all adequately represented. The overall estimate is more precise than that based on a simple random sample, which ignores the subgroup structure of the population. The usual strategy is to select the same proportion of individuals from each stratum (epsem scheme), that is to use the same **sampling fraction** for each stratum. It is sometimes necessary to adjust this, however, so that the sample sizes in very small strata are not too small.

Example 23.2
It was desired to estimate the prevalence rate of a disease in a country with three main geographical regions, coastal plain, mountainous, and semi-arid. As the population was not evenly spread throughout the country, and as it was thought that the geography might influence the prevalence rate of the disease, a stratified sample was chosen. Table 23.2 shows the results obtained with the estimated prevalence rates in each of the regions.

Table 23.2 Results from a stratified sample carried out to estimate the prevalence rate of a disease in a country with three main geographical regions. The overall prevalence rate is calculated by adding together the estimated total numbers of persons with the disease in each region, and dividing by the overall population*.

Region	Population	Sample size	Number diseased	Prevalence rate	Estimated total with disease
Coastal plain	1 500 000	200	120	0.6	900 000
Mountainous	150 000	50	5	0.1	15 000
Semi-arid	300 000	50	15	0.3	90 000
Total	1 950 000	300	140	*0.52	1 005 000

The overall prevalence rate is calculated by estimating the total numbers of individuals with the disease in each region. For example, in the coastal plain the sample prevalence rate was 120/200 or 0.6. Applying this to the total population living in the coastal plain gives an estimated number of $0.6 \times 1\,500\,000 = 900\,000$ persons with the disease. The numbers for the mountainous and semi-arid regions are similarly calculated and are 15 000 and 90 000 diseased persons respectively. The total number of diseased persons in the whole country is therefore estimated to be 1 005 000. The total population size is 1 950 000 and so the overall prevalence rate is estimated as $1\,005\,000/1\,950\,000 = 0.52$.

Note that this is not the same as the overall prevalence rate for the sample, which is 140/300 = 0.47. The two results agree only when the same sampling fraction has been used in each stratum (as was not the case here). The calculation of the standard error of the prevalence rate for the whole country is based on a combination of the standard errors of the estimated prevalences in each region. See Moser and Kalton (1971) or Cochran (1977) for the details.

Multi-stage sampling

Multi-stage sampling is carried out in stages using the hierarchical structure of a population. For example, a **two-stage sample** might consist of first taking a random sample of schools and then taking a random sample of children from each selected school. The schools would be called **first-stage units** and the children **second-stage units**. The advantages are that resources can be concentrated in a limited number of places and that a sampling frame is not needed for the whole population. A list of first-stage units is required, but second-stage units need only be listed for those first-stage units which are selected. The disadvantage is that the overall estimate is less precise than that based on a simple random sample of the same total size. In other words to achieve the same precision as a simple random sample requires a larger total sample size.

Sampling at the second stage consists of taking simple random samples of the same size from each of the selected first-stage units. The method of sampling the first-stage units depends on whether or not they all contain the same number of second-stage units. If they do, a simple random sample is taken. If they are of different sizes, an equal probability scheme is achieved by sampling with **probability proportional to size (p.p.s.)**. For example, if one school has twice as many pupils as another it is given twice the chance of being selected. p.p.s. sampling is performed **with replacement**, which means that after selection a first-stage unit is still included in the draw and may be selected again. When a first-stage unit is selected twice, twice the number of second-stage units are sampled from it. The overall effect is to give each second-stage unit in the population an equal chance of being selected.

It is also possible to have a scheme with more than two levels of sampling, for example selecting towns, districts, streets, and finally houses. This is called **multi-stage sampling**.

Cluster sampling

If very little extra cost is involved, it may be advisable to investigate all the second-stage units from each selected first-stage unit in a two-stage sampling scheme, rather than only a sample of them. This is referred to as **cluster sampling**, and the first-stage units are called **clusters** in this context. An equal probability scheme is achieved by taking a simple random sample of clusters regardless of whether or not they are all of the same size.

Cluster sampling is also preferred if some benefit is being offered to the participants which it would be ethically or logistically inappropriate to offer only to some members of the unit. For example, in sampling schools to estimate the prevalence rate of a disease when an effective treatment is to be offered to those found ill, it would be preferable to examine all pupils in the selected schools rather than just a sample of them.

Example 23.3

The stratified sample proposed in Example 23.2 to estimate the prevalence rate of a disease in a country with three main regions could be refined to sample first communities (towns, villages, or hamlets) and then houses in each region, examining all members of selected households. The resulting scheme would be a combination of stratified sampling (regions), two-stage sampling (communities and houses) and cluster sampling (all members of households).

CHAPTER 24

Cohort and Case–Control Studies

Introduction

The relative advantages and disadvantages of the case–control approach as compared to the cohort (or longitudinal) approach have already been discussed in Chapter 21. A cohort study involves follow-up of individuals from the determination of exposure status to the subsequent occurrence of disease. In contrast, a case–control study starts with the disease status of an individual and looks backward in time to determine the past exposure status to the risk factors of interest. For this reason, the terms **prospective** and **retrospective** are often used interchangeably with cohort and case–control respectively. This use of terminology is misleading, however, and is not recommended since, as mentioned in Chapter 21, it is occasionally possible to carry out a cohort study entirely retrospectively from past records.

In this chapter we focus on the measures of association used to assess the strength of the relationship between a risk factor and the subsequent occurrence of disease. Case–control studies are most easily understood by appreciating that behind every case–control study lies an equivalent cohort study. We therefore start by considering cohort studies.

Cohort studies

In a cohort study a sample of individuals, some exposed to the risk factor of interest and some not, are followed over time, and the rates of subsequently contracting the disease in the two groups are compared. For example, Table 24.1 shows some hypothetical data from a cohort study to investigate the association between smoking and lung cancer. Thirty thousand smokers and 60 000 non-smokers were followed for a year, during which time 39 of the smokers and six of the non-smokers developed lung cancer, giving incidence rates of 1.30 and 0.10 per 1000 per year respectively. Thus the incidence of lung cancer was considerably higher among smokers than non-smokers. In fact it was 13.0 (1.30/0.10) times higher. This ratio is called the **relative risk** and summarizes the strength of the association between the factor and the disease.

Table 24.1 Hypothetical data from a cohort study to investigate the association between smoking and lung cancer. The calculations of relative and attributable risk are illustrated.

	Lung cancer	No lung cancer	Total	Incidence rate
Smokers	39	29 961	30 000	1.30/1000/yr
Non-smokers	6	59 994	60 000	0.10/1000/yr
Total	45	89 955	90 000	

$RR = \frac{1.30}{0.10} = 13.0$, $AR = 1.30 - 0.10$, $= 1.20/1000/\text{yr}$ (smokers) $\quad$ Prop $AR = \frac{1.20}{1.30} = 0.923$ or 92.3%

Relative risk

$$\text{Relative risk (RR)} = \frac{\text{incidence among exposed}}{\text{incidence among non-exposed}}$$

A relative risk of 1 occurs when the incidences are the same in the two groups and is equivalent to no association between the risk factor and the disease. A relative risk greater than 1 occurs when the risk of disease is higher among those exposed to the factor than among the non-exposed, as in the above example with exposed referring to smoking. A relative risk less than 1 occurs when the risk is lower among those exposed, suggesting that the factor may be protective. An example is the reduced risk of diarrhoeal disease observed among infants that are breast-fed compared to those that are not. The further the relative risk is from 1, the stronger the association. Its statistical significance can be tested using a 2×2 χ^2 test, described in Chapter 13.

Confidence interval for RR

The calculation of the confidence interval is complicated. The formula given here is that due to Miettinen. It is a test-based approximation which means that it is calculated using the χ^2 value (in fact, its square root) found in the significance test, rather than a standard error.

$$95\% \text{ c.i.} = RR^{(1 \pm 1.96/\chi)}$$

Other percentage confidence intervals are obtained by replacing 1.96 with the appropriate percentage point of the normal distribution.

For example, consider the data presented in Table 24.1:

$$\text{RR} = 13.0, \quad \chi^2 = 55.25, \quad P < 0.001$$

Therefore

$$\chi = \sqrt{55.25} = 7.43 \text{ and } 1.96/\chi = 1.96/7.43 = 0.26$$

giving

$$\text{RR}^{(1+1.96/\chi)} = 13.0^{1+0.26} = 13.0^{1.26} = 25.3$$

and

$$\text{RR}^{(1-1.96/\chi)} = 13.0^{1-0.26} = 13.0^{0.74} = 6.7$$

The 95% confidence interval for the relative risk is therefore 6.7 to 25.3.

Attributable risk

The relative risk assesses how much more likely, for example, a smoker is to develop lung cancer than a non-smoker, but it gives no indication of the magnitude of the excess risk in absolute terms. This is measured by the **attributable risk**.

$$\begin{array}{c}\text{Attributable risk}\\ \text{(AR)}\end{array} = \begin{array}{c}\text{incidence}\\ \text{among exposed}\end{array} - \begin{array}{c}\text{incidence}\\ \text{among non-exposed}\end{array}$$

Attributable risk is sometimes expressed as a proportion (or percentage) of the total incidence rate among the exposed, and is then called the **proportional attributable risk**, the attributable proportion (exposed), the attributable fraction (exposed) or the aetiologic fraction (exposed).

$$\begin{array}{c}\text{Proportional}\\ \text{attributable risk}\end{array} = \frac{\begin{array}{c}\text{incidence}\\ \text{among exposed}\end{array} - \begin{array}{c}\text{incidence}\\ \text{among non-exposed}\end{array}}{\text{incidence among exposed}} = \frac{\text{RR}-1}{\text{RR}}$$

In the example, the attributable risk of lung cancer due to smoking was 1.30–0.10 = 1.20 cases per 1000 per year, with smoking accounting for 92.3% (1.20/1.30) of all the cases of lung cancer among the smokers.

Table 24.2 Relative and attributable risks of death from selected causes, 1951–1961, associated with heavy cigarette smoking by British male physicians. Data from Doll & Hill (1964) *British Medical Journal* **1,** 1399–1410, as presented by MacMahon & Pugh (1970) *Epidemiology—Principles and Methods.* Little, Brown & Co., Boston (with permission).

	Age-standardized death rate (per 1000 person–years)			
Cause of death	Non-smokers	Heavy smokers	RR	AR
Lung cancer	0.07	2.27	32.4	2.20
Other cancers	1.91	2.59	1.4	0.68
Chronic bronchitis	0.05	1.06	21.2	1.01
Cardiovascular disease	7.32	9.93	1.4	2.61
All causes	12.06	19.67	1.6	7.61

Table 24.2 shows the relative and attributable risks of death from selected causes associated with heavy cigarette smoking. The association has been most clearly demonstrated for lung cancer and chronic bronchitis, with relative risks of 32.4 and 21.2 respectively. If, however, the association with cardiovascular disease, although not so strong, is also accepted as being causative, elimination of smoking would save even more deaths due to cardiovascular disease than due to lung cancer, 2.61 compared to 2.20 for every 1000 smoker–years at risk. Note that the death rates were age-standardized to take account of the differing age distributions of smokers and non-smokers, and of the increase in death rates with age (*see* Chapter 15).

In summary, the relative risk is the best measure of the strength of an association between a risk factor and a disease. The larger its size, the more likely it is that the association is causal. The attributable risk, on the other hand, gives a better idea of the excess risk of disease experienced by an individual as the result of being exposed. The overall impact of the risk factor on the population also depends, however, on how prevalent exposure is. In population terms a rare exposure with a high associated relative risk may be less serious in the total number (or proportion) of deaths that it will cause than a very common exposure with a lower associated relative risk. This is assessed by the excess overall incidence in the population as compared with the incidence among the non-exposed. The resulting measure is the **population attributable risk**.

$$\text{Population attributable risk} = \text{overall incidence} - \text{incidence among non-exposed}$$

This may also be expressed as a proportion (or percentage) of the overall incidence. The resulting measure is the **population proportional attributable risk**, alternatively named the aetiologic fraction (population) or the attributable fraction (population).

$$\text{Population proportional attributable risk} = \frac{\text{overall incidence} - \text{incidence among non-exposed}}{\text{overall incidence}}$$

$$= \frac{\text{prevalence}_{\text{exposure}}(\text{RR}-1)}{1+\text{prevalence}_{\text{exposure}}(\text{RR}-1)}$$

Incidence rate, incidence risk, and odds ratio

Recall from Chapter 15 that incidence may be measured either as a risk or as a rate. The calculation of the risk is based on the population at risk at the start of the study, while the rate is based on the total person–years at risk (pyar) during the study and reflects the changing population at risk. This is illustrated for a cohort study in Figure 24.1, which shows the gradual accumulation of cases from those initially disease-free among the exposed and the non-exposed populations.

An alternative measure of incidence is the **odds** of disease to non-disease. This equals the total number of cases divided by those still at risk at the end of the study. Using the notation shown in Table 24.3 the odds among the exposed is a/b and among the non-exposed c/d. Their ratio is called the **odds ratio**. It equals:

$$\frac{a/b}{c/d} = \frac{ad}{bc}$$

which is the cross-product of the table. The odds ratio estimated from Table 24.1 equals $(39 \times 59994)/(6 \times 29961) = 13.0$.

$$\text{Odds ratio (OR)} = ad/bc$$

The odds ratio may equivalently be considered as the ratio of the odds of exposure to non-exposure among the diseased (a/c) compared to the non-diseased (b/d). For this reason it plays an important role in case–control studies (*see below*).

For a **rare disease**, that is one for which the proportion of cases in the population is very low, the lines in Figure 24.1 showing the accumulation of

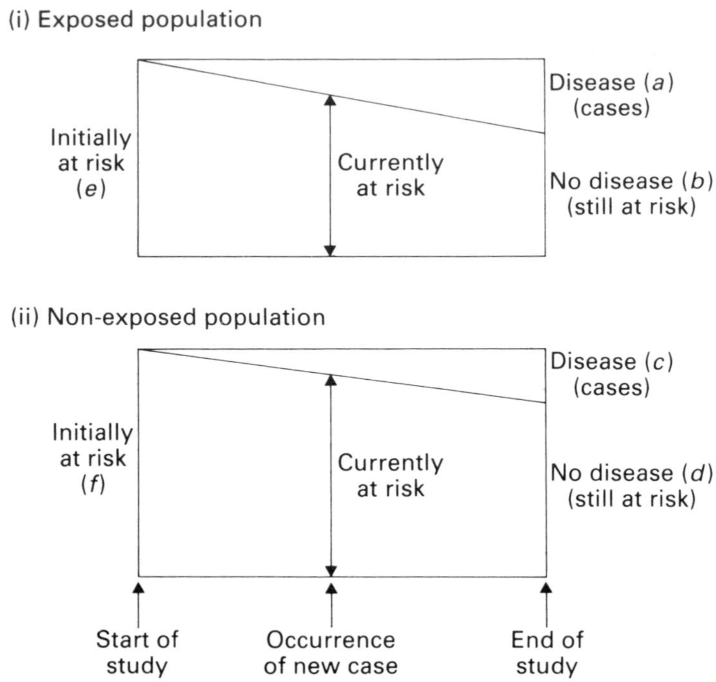

Figure 24.1 A graphical representation of a cohort study. The three possible measures of relative incidence are:

Relative risk (using incidence risks) $= \dfrac{a/e}{c/f}$

Relative risk (using incidence rates) $= \dfrac{\text{a/(pyar exposed)}}{c/\text{(pyar non-exposed)}}$

Odds ratio $= \dfrac{a/b}{c/d}$

cases will be almost horizontal and indistinguishable from the top lines representing the total populations under study. In this case *the three measures, incidence risk, incidence rate, and odds of disease, are numerically equal.*

Table 24.3 Notation for cohort and unmatched case–control studies.

	Disease	No disease	Total
Exposed	*a*	*b*	*e*
Non-exposed	*c*	*d*	*f*
Total	*g*	*h*	*n*

For a **common disease**, however, *the three measures are different*, and will lead to three different measures of association between factor and disease, the relative risk using incidence risks, the relative risk using incidence rates, and the odds ratio. The usual choice is to use incidence rates. The use of incidence risks is more appropriate, however, when assessing the protective effect of an exposure, such as a vaccine, which it is believed offers full protection to some individuals but none to others, rather than partial protection to all (Smith *et al.* 1984). The odds ratio is used in case–control studies (*see below*).

Case–control studies

In a case–control study, the sampling is carried out according to disease rather than exposure status. A group of individuals identified as having the disease, the **cases**, is compared with a group of individuals not having the disease, the **controls**, with respect to their prior exposure to the factor of interest. No information is obtained directly about the incidences in the exposed and non-exposed populations, but it can be shown that the cross-product ratio of the case–control table estimates the odds ratio. For a *rare* disease, this is numerically equivalent to the relative risk.

Table 24.4 shows the results from a case–control study to investigate the association between coffee drinking and cancer of the pancreas. A relative risk of 2.5 was obtained, suggesting that women who drink coffee are 2.5 times more likely to develop cancer of the pancreas than those who do not.

Rare disease: $\text{OR} = ad/bc = \text{RR}$
Common disease: $\text{OR} = ad/bc; \quad 0 < |\text{RR}| < |\text{OR}|$

For a *common* disease the meaning of the cross-product ratio depends on the sampling scheme used for controls (Smith *et al.* 1984). The most usual

Table 24.4 Results of a case–control study to investigate the association between coffee drinking and cancer of the pancreas. Data for women are shown. With permission from MacMahon *et al.* (1981) *New England Journal of Medicine* **304,** 630–3.

Coffee drinking	Cases	Controls	Total
Yes	140	280	420
No	11	56	67
Total	151	336	487

$$\text{OR} = \frac{140 \times 56}{11 \times 280} = 2.5$$

choice is to select controls from those still disease-free at the end of the study (the denominator group in the odds measure of incidence); any controls selected during the course of the study who subsequently develop disease are treated as cases and not as controls. In this case it can be shown that the cross-product ratio represents the odds ratio, and that the magnitude of the odds ratio, |OR|, is greater than that of the relative risk.

Confounding variables

In the design and analysis of a case–control study it is important to ensure that there are no confounding variables which may cause bias in investigating the association of interest. For example, in the study of coffee drinking and cancer of the pancreas, it would be necessary to ensure that the age distributions of the cases and controls were similar, as the risk of cancer of the pancreas is age-related. This could be arranged at the design stage either by selecting equal numbers of cases and controls from each age group (**stratum matching**) or by using a matched design (*see below*). Alternatively, it is possible to take confounding variables into account during the analysis, for example by subdividing the data into the different age-groups and calculating an odds ratio for each. An overall estimate is obtained by calculating ad/n and bc/n from each table. The ad/n's are then added up and divided by the sum of the bc/n's. This is called the Mantel–Haenszel estimate of the odds ratio, and the appropriate significance test is the Mantel–Haenszel summary χ^2 test (*see* Chapter 14).

$$\text{OR}_{\text{Mantel}-\text{Haenszel}} = \frac{\Sigma ad/n}{\Sigma bc/n}$$

A more sophisticated approach is to use logistic regression (*see* Chapter 14), and to estimate the odds ratio from the regression coefficients. This is appropriate for controlling simultaneously for several confounding variables, when the number of subsets required is large and when the numbers of individuals in each are likely to be very small. For details see Breslow and Day (1980) or Schlesselman (1982).

Matched designs

In a matched design, each case is matched with one or more controls, which are deliberately chosen to have the same values for any potential confounding variables. For example, Table 24.5 shows data from a study to investigate the association between use of oral contraceptives and thromboembolism. The

Table 24.5 Results of a case–control study with *matched* data to investigate the association between use of oral contraceptives (OC) and thromboembolism. With permission from Sartwell *et al.* (1969) *American Journal of Epidemiology* **90,** 365–80.

		Controls		
		OC used	OC not used	Total
Cases	OC used	10	57	67
	OC not used	13	95	108
	Total	23	152	175

$$OR = \frac{57}{13} = 4.4$$

cases were 175 women aged 15–44 discharged alive from 43 hospitals after initial attacks of thromboembolism. For each case a female patient suffering from some other disease (thought to be unrelated to the use of oral contraceptives) was selected from the same hospital to act as a control. She was chosen to have the same residence, time of hospitalization, race, age, marital status, parity, and income status as the case. Participants were questionned about their past contraceptive history, and in particular about whether they had used oral contraceptives during the month before they were admitted to hospital.

The pairing of the cases and controls is preserved in the analysis by tabulating oral contraceptive use of the case against oral contraceptive use of the control. There were 10 case–control pairs in which both case and control had used oral contraceptives and 95 pairs in which neither had. These 105 pairs give no information about the association. This information is entirely contained in the 70 pairs in which the case and control differed. There were 57 case–control pairs in which only the case had used oral contraceptives within the previous month compared to 13 in which only the control had done so. The odds ratio is measured by the ratio of these **discordant pairs** and equals 4.4 (=57/13). The appropriate significance test is McNemar's χ^2 test for the comparison of paired proportions (*see* Chapter 14), which gives $\chi^2 = 26.4$, $P < 0.001$.

OR = ratio of discordant pairs

$$= \frac{\text{no. of pairs in which case exposed, control not exposed}}{\text{no. of pairs in which control exposed, case not exposed}}$$

If *several* controls rather than a single matched control are selected for each case, the odds ratio is estimated using a special application of the Mantel–Haenszel procedures. Finally, the analysis of several risk factors, or the need to adjust for confounding variables additional to those matched for in the design, requires a special form of logistic regression called **conditional logistic regression**. The different methods of analysis are summarized in Table

Table 24.6 Analysis of case–control studies—summary of methods.

Sampling scheme for controls	Single risk factor	Several risk factors / adjustment for confounding variables
(a) *One control per case*		
Random	Simple 2×2 table showing risk factor $\times$ case/control Standard χ^2 test OR = cross-product ratio, ad/bc	Logistic regression or stratified analysis
Pairwise matching	2×2 table showing agreement between cases and controls with respect to risk factor McNemar's χ^2 test OR = ratio of discordant pairs $= \frac{\text{case yes, control no}}{\text{case no, control yes}}$	Conditional logistic regression
Stratum matching	Stratified analysis: 2×2 table for each stratum Mantel–Haenszel χ^2 test $\text{OR} = \frac{\Sigma(ad/n)}{\Sigma(bc/n)}$	Logistic regression or stratified analysis
(b) *Multiple controls per case*		
Random	As above	As above
Matched sets of each case and its associated controls	Special application of Mantel–Haenszel procedures	Conditional logistic regression
Stratum matching	As above	As above
(c) *Confidence intervals*		
All schemes	$95\% = \text{OR}^{(1 \pm 1.96/\chi)}$ Miettinen's test-based approximation	Calculate from regression coefficients

24.6. For full discussion of these more complicated situations, consult Breslow and Day (1980) or Schlesselman (1982).

Confidence interval for the odds ratio

The confidence interval for the odds ratio can be calculated in the same way as that for the relative risk, using Miettinen's test-based approach.

$$95\% \text{ c.i.} = \text{OR}^{(1 \pm 1.96/\chi)}$$

Other percentage confidence intervals are obtained by replacing 1.96 with the appropriate percentage point of the normal distribution. This formula applies whether the χ^2 test used was the standard 2×2 table version, the Mantel–Haenszel test or McNemar's paired test. In all instances, the square root of the χ^2 value is taken.

For example, consider the matched data presented in Table 24.5 on the association between oral contraceptive use and thromboembolism, for which:

$$\text{OR} = 4.4, \quad \chi^2 = 26.4, \quad P < 0.001$$

Therefore:

$$\chi = \sqrt{26.4} = 5.14 \quad \text{and} \quad 1.96/\chi = 1.96/5.14 = 0.38$$

giving

$$\text{OR}^{(1+1.96/\chi)} = 4.4^{1+0.38} = 4.4^{1.38} = 7.7$$

and

$$\text{OR}^{(1-1.96/\chi)} = 4.4^{1-0.38} = 4.4^{0.62} = 2.5$$

The 95% confidence interval for the odds ratio is therefore 2.5 to 7.7.

CHAPTER 25

Clinical Trials and Intervention Studies

Introduction

The three categories of experimental studies (clinical, vaccine, and intervention trials) were briefly introduced in Chapter 21. Their main design features will now be described. For simplicity, the discussion will focus on clinical trials, but it will apply equally to trials of prophylactic regimes or preventive measures. Features relating specifically to vaccine and other intervention trials will be considered briefly at the end of the chapter. For a comprehensive discussion of clinical trials see Pocock (1983).

Clinical trials

A clinical trial is an experiment carried out to assess the effectiveness of a new treatment regime. Volunteers are allocated to one of two groups, the **treatment group** or the **control group**. The control group receives either the standard treatment for the condition, as in the evaluation of a new drug, or no effective treatment, as in the assessment of the efficacy of a vaccine. Extensions of the method are the inclusion of several different dosage groups and the simultaneous trial of several different treatment regimes.

It is important to design the trial so that any observed difference between the treatment and control groups can be attributed to a real effect of the treatment. The groups should initially be as alike as possible in all respects other than the treatment received. It would be no good if, for example, the control group initially contained relatively more persons with a severe condition than the treatment group, since this alone would make the treatment appear effective. In other words, care must be taken to avoid *selection bias*. This is accomplished by the use of *randomization*, sometimes augmented by a *matched* or *cross-over design*.

Furthermore, the methods of handling and assessing the groups should be the same. The opportunity for any bias to occur during the conduct of the trial is minimized by the use of a *single-* or *double-blind* designs and a *placebo*.

Randomization

Random allocation of participants to the treatment and control groups is the method used to avoid any bias in selection (conscious or otherwise), either by the investigators or by the participants, which may lead to inherent differences between the groups. This is most conveniently carried out using random number tables (*see* Chapter 23). One-digit numbers are selected, with odd numbers (1, 3, 5, 7, 9) corresponding to the treatment group and even numbers (0, 2, 4, 6, 8) to the control group (or vice versa). Suppose the first six selected numbers were 2, 7, 9, 0, 4, 7, then the first participant would be allocated to the control group, the second and the third to the treatment group, the fourth and fifth to the control group, and the sixth to the treatment group.

It is sometimes desirable to arrange the allocations so that after every 10, for example, equal numbers of participants have been entered into each group. This is called **restricted randomization** or **randomization with balance**. In this case the use of the tables is slightly different. For each set of 10 participants, for example, the tables are used to decide which five will be allocated to the treatment group by selecting five different numbers between 01 and 10. Suppose 09, 02, 04, 01, 08 are chosen. Then the first, second, fourth, eighth and ninth participants of the set will be allocated to the treatment group and the others, that is the third, fifth, sixth, seventh and tenth, will be allocated to the control group. This randomization procedure is repeated for each set of 10 participants.

Randomization may also be modified to ensure, for example, the same proportion of males and females in each group, by using separate random allocation series for each sex.

The order of allocation should preferably be decided before the start of the trial. It is recommended that a set of numbered envelopes containing the allocations is prepared, to be opened in order as each new person is accepted into the trial.

Matching

Alternatively, a **matched-pair design** may be used to arrange explicitly that the treatment and control groups are similar for the main confounding variables, such as age and sex. Participants are paired according to the matching variables, and one member of each pair is then allocated at random to the treatment group, and the other to the control group. Note that this matching should be preserved in the analysis, for example by carrying out McNemar's χ^2 test (*see* Chapter 14) rather than the standard 2×2 χ^2 test.

A matched-pair design is less suitable than straightforward randomization when there is a gradual entry of participants to the trial taking place over an extended period of time as there may be considerable delay before a suitable match is found for a new participant.

Cross-over design

In a clinical trial of a regime offering relatively short-term benefits, it may be appropriate to use participants as their own controls. For example, in the comparison of two analgesics (A and B) for treatment of migraine each participant could try each of the preparations on different occasions. The order of use of the preparations should be randomized, so that half the participants try analgesic A first, and the other half try analgesic B first. This is called a **cross-over design**. The main disadvantage is the possibility of a residual or **spill-over effect** from the first occasion affecting the result of the second.

Single- and double-blind designs

Whenever possible it is preferable that neither the participant nor the investigator knows which treatment has been received until after the end of the trial. This is called a **double-blind design** and ensures against biases in the handling or assessment of the groups. It is particularly necessary if any *subjective* assessments are involved. To achieve this the therapy given to the control group must be made indistinguishable in appearance to that given to the treatment group. This may entail the use of a **placebo** preparation with no effective action for the control group. The treatment and control preparations are identified by code alone, the code being held by an uninterested party until all the data have been collected. A **single-blind design** is when the investigator but not the participant knows the treatment received.

Ethical issues

Although scientifically a randomized controlled trial is the best way to demonstrate the benefit of a treatment regime, its use raises important ethical issues. Is it justified to withhold a treatment from the control group that might be beneficial to them? This is particularly relevant when the new treatment is believed unlikely to have any adverse side-effects and there is either no standard treatment or no efficacious standard treatment. An example of this is the suggestion that vitamin supplements during pregnancy may reduce the incidence of neural tube defects. Also, is randomization justified, or should participants be able to choose which group they are in? Is informed consent necessary? This is well discussed in the context of lumpectomy or mastectomy for treating breast cancer by the Cancer Research Campaign Working Party in Breast Conservation (1983). For a fuller discussion of these and related issues see Bradford Hill (1977) who also includes copies of the Medical Research Council's Statement on Responsibility in Investigations on Human Subjects and of the Helsinki Declaration of the World Medical Assembly on Recommendations Guiding Medical Doctors in Biomedical Research Involving Human Subjects.

Sequential clinical trials

A sequential clinical trial is one in which the results are assessed continuously in order to see whether sufficient evidence has accumulated to stop the trial and to claim *either* that a difference has been demonstrated *or* that there is no difference.

Sequential trials are most commonly used when the outcome measure is a proportion, such as the proportion surviving in each of the two treatment groups. The methodology will be illustrated by considering a specific example. (For more details see Armitage, 1975.) Figure 25.1 shows the results of a

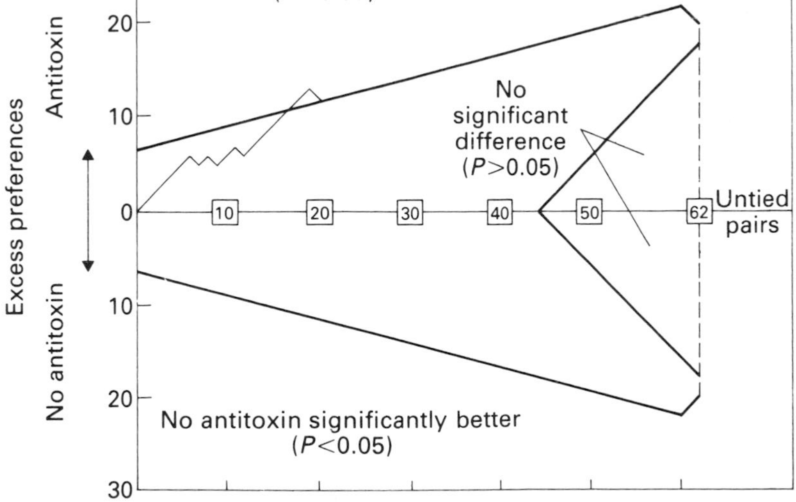

Figure 25.1 Results from a sequential trial to assess the value of a large dose of antitoxin in treating clinical tetanus. With permission from Brown *et al.* (1960) Lancet **ii**, 227–30

trial to assess the effectiveness of a large dose of antitoxin in treating clinical tetanus by comparing mortality rates among those who were and who were not given antitoxin. Participants were arranged in pairs, one of whom received the antitoxin and one of whom did not. If the member of the pair receiving antitoxin survived while the other died this was a preference in favour of the antitoxin. Conversely, if the member receiving antitoxin died while the other survived this was a preference in favour of no antitoxin. If both members of the pair either survived or died, this was a tied pair and contributed no information to the comparison of antitoxin with no antitoxin.

The results were recorded as obtained on a graph showing the number of excess preferences against the number of untied pairs. The plot started at zero and was drawn one unit up and to the right for each preference in favour of antitoxin and one unit down and to the right for each preference in favour of no antitoxin. The upper and lower boundaries were drawn to represent a result significant at the 5% level, and to give a 95% chance of one or other line being crossed if the rate of excess preferences was 75% or more. The middle wedge-shaped lines represented no significant difference. The upper boundary was crossed at the 18th preference and the trial stopped. Fifteen pairs gave survival results in favour of antitoxin and three in favour of no antitoxin, thus demonstrating a significantly lower mortality among those given antitoxin ($P<0.05$).

The main advantage of a sequential clinical trial is that, on average, fewer participants are needed to arrive at a conclusion than in a fixed size trial where the analysis is carried out just once, at completion. This is balanced, however, against a generally lower level of significance being obtained since adjustment is made, when drawing the boundaries, for the increased likelihood of a chance significant result due to the repeated testing. Thus, in the above example the significance level obtained was 5%. Without the adjustment, McNemar's test (*see* Chapter 14) yields a χ^2 value of 6.7 for the comparison of 15 out of 18 pairs in favour of antitoxin with only three in favour of no antitoxin. This is significant at the 1% level. A practical consideration is that sequential trials are not appropriate for the many situations where there is a long time interval between the administration of the treatment and the final assessment of the response under study.

Vaccine trials

The design issues of a vaccine trial are exactly analogous to those of clinical trials of drugs (or other therapeutic measures), and a randomized controlled design is preferred. The objectives of a vaccine trial are, however, completely different. Vaccination is a preventive measure and the vaccine and its placebo are administered to healthy individuals rather than to ill persons. The aim is to assess the **efficacy** of the vaccination in preventing the occurrence of disease. This is measured as the proportion of the cases in the placebo group that would not have occurred had they received vaccination.

For example, consider Table 25.1 which presents the results from a trial of a new influenza vaccine. A total of 80 cases of influenza occurred in the placebo group. If this group had instead received vaccination one would have expected only 8.3% (the rate experienced by the vaccinated group) of them to have developed influenza, that is $220 \times 0.083 = 18.3$ cases. The saving would therefore have been $80 - 18.3 = 61.7$ cases, giving a vaccine efficacy of $61.7/80 = 77\%$.

Table 25.1 Results from an influenza vaccine trial, previously presented in Table 13.1.

Influenza	Vaccine	Placebo	Total
Yes	20 (8.3%)	80 (36.4%)	100 (21.7%)
No	220	140	360
Total	240	220	460

This calculation can be simplified to the following formula, which more clearly shows the link between vaccine efficacy and relative risk associated with non-vaccination.

$$\text{Vaccine efficacy (VE)} = 1 - \frac{\text{incidence of disease in vaccinated}}{\text{incidence of disease in unvaccinated}} = 1 - \frac{1}{\text{RR}}$$

This formula is also used as the basis for calculation of a confidence interval for vaccine efficacy. A confidence interval for relative risk is first computed, as described in Chapter 24. The confidence limits are then inserted into this formula to give the corresponding limits for vaccine efficacy.

$$95\%\ \text{c.i.}\,(\text{VE}) = 1 - \frac{1}{\text{RR}^{1 \pm 1.96/\chi}}$$

In this example,

$$RR = \frac{80/220}{20/240} = 4.36; \quad VE = 1 - \frac{1}{RR} = 1 - \frac{1}{4.36} = 0.77 \text{ (as above)}$$

$$\chi^2 = 51.37 \text{ and therefore } \chi = \sqrt{51.37} = 7.17$$

Lower confidence limit:

$$RR^{1-1.96/7.17} = 4.36^{1-0.27} = 4.36^{0.73} = 2.93$$

Corresponding $VE = 1 - 1/2.93 = 0.66$

Upper confidence limit:

$$RR^{1+1.96/7.17} = 3.36^{1+0.27} = 4.36^{1.27} = 6.49$$

Corresponding $VE = 1 - 1/6.49 = 0.85$

Thus the 95% confidence interval for vaccine efficacy for this influenza vaccine is between 66% and 85%.

Intervention studies

Intervention trials are the other main category of experimental studies. Their basic design is similar to that of a clinical trial, with one major exception. The application of the intervention is often (although not always) applied at the community rather than at the individual level. Examples are the assessment of the effect on dental caries of introducing fluoride into the drinking water of some districts and not others, and the evaluation of the impact on the incidence of diarrhoeal disease of an improved water supply. The particular issues that such community-based trials raise is a relatively neglected area and is beyond the scope of this book (*see* Smith, 1987).

CHAPTER 26

Calculation of Required Sample Size

Introduction

An essential part of planning any investigation is to decide how many people need to be studied in order to answer the study objectives. Too often the number is just pulled out of a hat, or decided on purely logistic grounds. This is bad practice, and considered by many to be unethical. On the one hand, studying many more persons than strictly necessary is a waste of time, money and (usually limited) resources. In a clinical trial, for example, this would not only mean that more persons than necessary were given the placebo, but that the introduction of the beneficial therapy it demonstrated was delayed. On the other hand, embarking on a study too small to be able to answer its objectives is equally questionable.

Calculating the required sample size is, however, not always a straightforward procedure as it first requires quantifying the objectives. For example, it would not be sufficient to state simply that the objective is to demonstrate whether or not formula-fed infants are at greater risk of death than breast-fed ones. It would also be necessary to state the size of the increased risk that it was desired to demonstrate since, for example, a smaller study would be needed to detect a fourfold increase than a twofold one. Furthermore, whatever the size of the increase, because of sampling variation (*see* Chapter 3) there will always be a possibility that a very much smaller risk is observed, and so we cannot guarantee that the study will yield a significant result. What we can do is to specify the probability that we would like to have of achieving statistical significance, at say the 5% level. This probability is called the **power** of the study. Thus we might decide that the study would be worthwhile if there was a 90% probability of demonstrating a difference in risk of death between bottle and breast-fed infants if the true relative risk was as high as 2.

The principles involved in sample size determination will now be discussed by considering a simple example in detail. This will be followed by a general discussion. Finally, the different formulae required for the most common situations will be presented (Table 26.2) and their application illustrated.

Principles involved in sample size determination

In Chapter 12 we discussed the analysis of the results from a clinical trial to compare two analgesic drugs, in which nine out of 12 migraine sufferers stated that they received greater relief with drug A than with drug B. This excess proportion, 0.75, in favour of drug A, was not, however, significant ($P = 0.15$), showing that the result was consistent with the null hypothesis of no difference in effectiveness between the drugs. This could mean one of two things, *either* that there really is no difference between the drugs *or* that drug A is better but that the sample size of 12 was not large enough to show this.

Consider now the design of such a study, and how many patients we would need in order to be able to demonstrate the superiority of drug A. Firstly, we must be more specific about what we mean by superiority. We will start by stating this as an overall preference rate of 70% or more for drug A and we will decide that we would like a 90% power of achieving a significant result at the 5% level.

The principles behind sample size determination are best introduced by considering different possible sample sizes and assessing their adequacy in fulfilling our requirements. We will start with a sample size of 20, as depicted in Figure 26.1(a). Recall that a result is significant at the 5% level if it is 1.96 s.e. or more away from the mean, that the null hypothesis value for the proportion of preferences for drug A is 0.5, and that the standard error (s.e.) therefore equals $\sqrt{(0.5 \times 0.5/n)}$. What does this mean for a sample size of 20?

$$\text{s.e.} = \sqrt{(0.5 \times 0.5/20)} = 0.1118$$

$$0.5 + 1.96 \text{ s.e.} = 0.5 + 1.96 \times 0.1118 = 0.72$$

$$\text{and} \quad 0.5 - 1.96 \text{ s.e.} = 0.5 - 1.96 \times 0.1118 = 0.28$$

Thus the range of values that would lead to a significant result are 0.72 and above and 0.28 and below.

If the **true** proportion is 0.7, what is the likelihood of observing 0.72 or above, and thus getting a significant result? This is illustrated by the shaded area in the figure. The curve represents the sampling distribution, which is a normal distribution centred on 0.7 with a standard error of $\sqrt{(0.7 \times 0.3/20)} = 0.1025$. The z value corresponding to 0.72 is:

$$\frac{0.72 - 0.7}{0.1025} = 0.20$$

The proportion of the standard normal distribution above 0.20 is found from Table A1 to equal 0.421, or 42.1%. In summary therefore, this means that with a sample size of 20 we have only a 42.1% chance of demonstrating that drug A is better, if the true preference rate is 0.7.

Consider next what happens if we increase the sample size to 50, as shown in Figure 26.1(b). The ranges of values which would now be significant have widened to 0.64 and above and to 0.36 and below. The sampling distribution

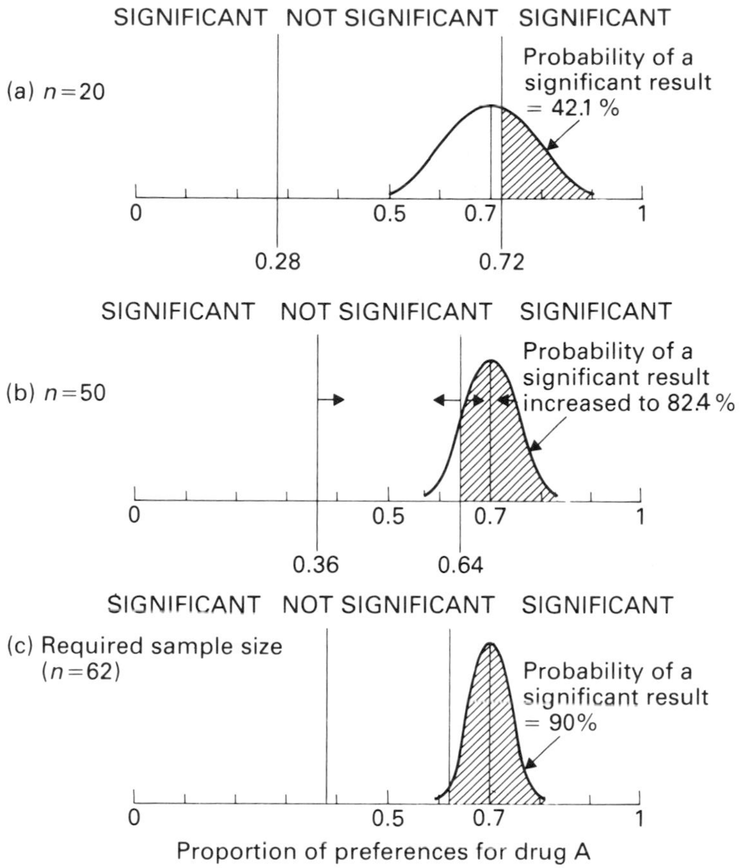

Figure 26.1 Probability of obtaining a significant result (at the 5% level) with various sample sizes (n) when testing the proportion of preferences for drug A rather than drug B against the null hypothesis value of 0.5, if the true value is 0.7

has narrowed, and there is a greater overlap with the significant ranges. Consequently, the probability of a significant result has increased. It is now found to be 82.4%, but this is still less than our required 90%.

Thus we certainly need to study more than 50 patients to have a 90% power. But how many more do we need? We need to increase the sample size, n, to the point where the overlap between the sampling distribution and the significant ranges reaches 90%, as shown in Figure 26.1(c). We will now describe how to calculate directly the sample size needed to do this. A significant result will be achieved if we observe a value above

$$0.5 + 1.96 \text{ s.e.} = 0.5 + 1.96 \times \sqrt{(0.5 \times 0.5/n)}$$

(or below $0.5 - 1.96$ s.e.). We want to select a large enough n so that 90% of the sampling distribution is above this point. The z value of the sampling distribution corresponding to 90% is -1.28 (*see* Table A2), which means an observed value of

$$0.7 - 1.28 \text{ s.e.} = 0.7 - 1.28 \times \sqrt{(0.7 \times 0.3/n)}$$

Therefore, n should be chosen large enough so that

$$0.7 - 1.28 \times \sqrt{(0.7 \times 0.3/n)} > 0.5 + 1.96 \times \sqrt{(0.5 \times 0.5/n)}$$

Rearranging this gives

$$0.7 - 0.5 > \frac{1.96 \times \sqrt{(0.5 \times 0.5)} + 1.28 \times \sqrt{(0.7 \times 0.3)}}{\sqrt{n}}$$

Squaring both sides, and further rearrangement gives

$$n > \frac{[1.96 \times \sqrt{(0.5 \times 0.5)} + 1.28 \times \sqrt{(0.7 \times 0.3)}]^2}{0.2^2}$$

$$= \frac{1.5666^2}{0.2^2} = 61.4$$

We therefore require about 60 patients to satisfy our requirements of having a 90% power of demonstrating a significant difference between drugs A and B at the 5% level, if the true preference rate for drug A was as high as 0.7.

Formulae for sample size calculations

The above discussion related to sample size determination for a significance test of a single proportion, namely the proportion of participants preferring drug A to drug B. In practice it is not necessary to go through such detailed reasoning every time. Instead the sample size can be calculated directly from a general formula, which for the significance test of a single proportion is:

$$n > \frac{\{u\sqrt{[\pi(1-\pi)]} + v\sqrt{[\pi_0(1-\pi_0)]}\}^2}{(\pi - \pi_0)^2}$$

where

$n =$ required minimum sample size

$\pi =$ proportion of interest

$\pi_0 =$ null hypothesis proportion

$u =$ one-sided percentage point of the normal distribution corresponding to 100% − the power, e.g. if power = 90%, (100% − power) = 10% and $u = 1.28$

$v =$ percentage of the normal distribution corresponding to the required (two-sided) significance level, e.g. if significance level = 5%, $v = 1.96$

For example, in applying this formula to the above example we have:

$$\pi = 0.7, \quad \pi_0 = 0.5, \quad u = 1.28 \quad \text{and} \quad v = 1.96$$

giving

$$n > \frac{[1.28 \times \sqrt{(0.7 \times 0.3)} + 1.96 \times \sqrt{(0.5 \times 0.5)}]^2}{(0.7 - 0.5)^2}$$

$$= \frac{1.5666^2}{0.2^2} = 61.4$$

which is exactly the same as obtained above.

The same principles can also be applied in other cases. Detailed reasoning is not given here but the appropriate formulae for use in the most common situations are listed in Table 26.1. The list consists of two parts. Table 26.1(a) covers cases where the aim of the study is to demonstrate a significant difference. Table 26.1(b) covers situations where the aim is to estimate a quantity of interest with a specified precision. Note that for the cases with two means, proportions, or rates, the formulae give the sample sizes required for each of the two groups. The total size of the study is therefore twice this. Table 26.2 gives adjustment factors for *study designs with unequal size groups* (*see* Example 26.3). Note also that the formulae applying to rates give thc required sample size in the same unit as the rates (*see* Example 26.2).

The use of the table will be illustrated by several examples. It is important to realize that sample size calculations are based on our best guesses of a situation. The number arrived at is not magical. It simply gives an idea of the sort of numbers to be studied. In other words, it is useful for distinguishing between 50 and 100, but not between 51 and 52. For this reason, continuity corrections have not been included in the formulae relating to proportions, as this was considered an unnecessary complication to achieve more mathematical accuracy than needed. Furthermore, the guesses made are unlikely to be correct, since if we knew the answers we would not be needing to do the study. It is therefore essential to carry out sample size calculations for several different scenarios, not just one. This gives a clearer picture of the possible scope of the study and is helpful in weighing up the balance between what is desirable and what is logistically feasible.

Finally, the sample size should be increased to allow for possible non-response or loss to follow-up. Further adjustments should be made to allow for such things as the use of a cluster rather than basic random sampling scheme, and the need to control for confounding variables in the analysis. This is not only beyond the scope of this book, but also a relatively undeveloped area.

Table 26.1 Formulae for sample size determination. (a) For studies where the aim is to demonstrate a significant difference. (b) For studies where the aim is to estimate a quantity of interest with a specified precision.

		Information needed	Formula for minimum sample size
(a) *Significant result*			
1 Single mean	$\mu-\mu_0$	Difference between mean, μ, and null hypothesis value, μ_0	$\dfrac{(u+v)^2\sigma^2}{(\mu-\mu_0)^2}$
	σ	Standard deviation	
	u, v	As below	
2 Single rate*	μ	Rate	$\dfrac{(u+v)^2\mu}{(\mu-\mu_0)^2}$
	μ_0	Null hypothesis value	
	u, v	As below	
3 Single proportion	π	Proportion	$\dfrac{\{u\sqrt{[\pi(1-\pi)]}+v\sqrt{[\pi_0(1-\pi_0)]}\}^2}{(\pi-\pi_0)^2}$
	π_0	Null hypothesis value	
	u, v	As below	
4 Comparison of two means (sample size of each group)	$\mu_1-\mu_2$	Difference between the means	$\dfrac{(u+v)^2(\sigma_1^2+\sigma_2^2)}{(\mu_1-\mu_2)^2}$
	σ_1, σ_2	Standard deviations	
	u, v	As below	
5 Comparison of two rates* (sample size of each group)	μ_1, μ_2	Rates	$\dfrac{(u+v)^2(\mu_1+\mu_2)}{(\mu_1-\mu_2)^2}$
	u, v	As below	
6 Comparison of two proportions (sample size of each group)	π_1, π_2	Proportions	$\dfrac{\{u\sqrt{[\pi_1(1-\pi_1)+\pi_2(1-\pi_2)]}+v\sqrt{[2\bar{\pi}(1-\bar{\pi})]}\}^2}{(\pi_2-\pi_1)^2}$
	u, v	As below	
			where $\bar{\pi}=\dfrac{\pi_1+\pi_2}{2}$
7 Case–control study (sample size of each group)	π_1	Proportion of controls exposed	$\dfrac{\{u\sqrt{[\pi_1(1-\pi_1)+\pi_2(1-\pi_2)]}+v\sqrt{[2\bar{\pi}(1-\bar{\pi})]}\}^2}{(\pi_2-\pi_1)^2}$
	OR	Odds ratio	
	π_2	Proportion of cases exposed, calculated from $\pi_2=\dfrac{\pi_1\text{OR}}{1+\pi_1(\text{OR}-1)}$	where $\bar{\pi}=\dfrac{\pi_1+\pi_2}{2}$

	u, v	As below	
All cases	u	One-sided percentage point of the normal distribution corresponding to 100%—the power, e.g. if power = 90%, $u = 1.28$	
	v	Percentage point of the normal distribution corresponding to the (two-sided) significance level, e.g. if significance level = 5%, $v = 1.96$	
(b) *Precision*			
8 Single mean	σ e	Standard deviation Required size of standard error	$\dfrac{\sigma^2}{e^2}$
9 Single rate*	μ e	Rate Required size of standard error	$\dfrac{\mu}{e^2}$
10 Single proportion	π e	Proportion Required size of standard error	$\dfrac{\pi(1-\pi)}{e^2}$
11 Difference between two means (sample size of each group)	σ_1, σ_2 e	Standard deviations Required size of standard error	$\dfrac{\sigma_1^2+\sigma_2^2}{e^2}$
12 Difference between two rates* (sample size of each group)	μ_1, μ_2 e	Rates Required size of standard error	$\dfrac{\mu_1+\mu_2}{e^2}$
13 Difference between two proportions (sample size of each group)	π_1, π_2 e	Proportions Required size of standard error	$\dfrac{\pi_1(1-\pi_1)+\pi_2(1-\pi_2)}{e^2}$

* In these cases the sample size refers to the same units as used for the denominator of the rate(s). For example, if the rate is expressed per person–year, the formula gives the number of person–years of observation required (*see* Example 26.2).

Example 26.1

A study is to be carried out in a rural area of East Africa to ascertain whether giving food supplementation during pregnancy increases birth weight. Women attending the antenatal clinic are to be randomly assigned to either receive or not receive supplementation. Formula 4 in Table 26.1 will help us to decide how many women should be enrolled in each group. We need to supply the following information:

(a) The size of the difference between mean birth weights that we would like to be able to detect. After much consideration it was decided that an increase of 0.25 kg was an appreciable effect that we would not like to miss. We therefore need to apply the formula with $\mu_1 - \mu_2 = 0.25$ kg.

(b) The standard deviations of the distributions of birth weight in each group. It was decided to assume that the standard deviation of birth weight would be the same in the two groups. Past data suggested that it would be about 0.4 kg. In other words we decided to assume that $\sigma_1 = 0.4$ kg and $\sigma_2 = 0.4$ kg.

(c) The power required. 95% was agreed on. We therefore need $u = 1.64$.

(d) The significance level required. It was decided that if possible we would like to achieve a result significant at the 1% level. We therefore need $v = 2.58$.

Applying formula 4 with these values gives:

$$n > \frac{(1.64 + 2.58)^2 \times (0.4^2 + 0.4^2)}{0.25^2}$$

$$= \frac{17.8084 \times 0.32}{0.0625} = 91.2$$

Therefore, in order to satisfy our requirements, we would need to enrol about 90 women in each group.

Example 26.2

Before embarking on a major water supply, sanitation, and hygiene intervention in southern Bangladesh, we would first like to know the average number of episodes of diarrhoea per year experienced by under-5-year-olds. We guess that this incidence is probably about 3, but would like to estimate it within ± 0.2. This means that if, for example, we observed 2.6 episodes/child/year, we would like to be able to conclude that the true rate was probably between 2.4 and 2.8 episodes/child/year. Expressing this in more statistical terms, we would like our 95% confidence interval to be no wider than ± 0.2. As the width of this confidence interval is approximately ± 2 s.e.'s, this means that we would like to study enough children to give a standard error as small as 0.1 episodes/child/year. Applying formula 9 in Table 26.1

gives:

$$n > \frac{3}{0.1^2} = 300$$

Note that the formulae applying to rates (numbers 3, 6, 11, 14) give the required sample size in the same unit as the rates. We specified the rates as per child per year. We therefore need to study 300 child–years to yield the desired precision. This could be achieved by observing 300 children for one year each or, for example, by observing four times as many (1200) for 3 months each. It is important not to overlook, however, the possibility of other factors such as seasonal effects when deciding on the time interval for a study involving the measurement of incidence rates.

Example 26.3
A case–control study is planned to investigate whether bottle-fed infants are at increased risk of death from acute respiratory infections compared to breast-fed infants. The mothers of a group of cases (infant deaths, with an underlying respiratory cause named on the death certificate) will be interviewed about the breast-feeding status of the child prior to the illness leading to death. The results will be compared with those obtained from mothers of a group of healthy controls regarding the current breast-feeding status of their infants. It is expected that about 40% of controls ($\pi_1 = 0.4$) will be bottle-fed,

Table 26.2 Adjustment factor for use in study designs to compare unequal sized groups, such as in a case–control study selecting multiple controls per case. This factor (f) applies to the smaller group and equals $(c+1)/(2c)$, where the size of the larger group is to be c times that of the smaller group. The sample size of the smaller group is therefore fn, where n would be the number required for equal-sized groups, and that of the larger group is cfn (*see* Example 26.3).

Ratio of larger to smaller group (c)	Adjustment to sample size of smaller group (f)
1	1
2	3/4
3	2/3
4	5/8
5	3/5
6	7/12
7	4/7
8	9/16
9	5/9
10	11/20

and we would like to detect a difference if bottle-feeding was associated with a twofold increase of death (OR = 2). How many cases and controls need to be studied to give a 90% power ($u = 1.28$) of achieving 5% significance ($v = 1.96$)? The calculation consists of several steps as detailed in formula 7 of Table 26.1.

(a) Calculate π_2, the proportion of cases bottle-fed:

$$\pi_2 = \frac{\pi_1 \text{OR}}{1 + \pi_1(\text{OR} - 1)} = \frac{0.4 \times 2}{1 + 0.4 \times (2 - 1)} = \frac{0.8}{1.4} = 0.57$$

(b) Calculate $\bar{\pi}$, the average of π_1 and π_2:

$$\bar{\pi} = \frac{0.4 + 0.57}{2} = 0.485$$

(c) Calculate the minimum sample size:

$$n > \frac{[1.28\sqrt{(0.4 \times 0.6 + 0.57 \times 0.43)} + 1.96\sqrt{(2 \times 0.485 \times 0.515)}]^2}{(0.57 - 0.4)^2}$$

$$= \frac{[1.28\sqrt{0.4851} + 1.96\sqrt{0.4996}]^2}{0.17^2} = \frac{2.2769^2}{0.17^2} = 179.4$$

We would therefore need to recruit about 180 cases and 180 controls, giving a total sample size of 360. What difference would it make if, rather than recruiting equal numbers of cases and controls, we decided to recruit three times as many controls as cases. Table 26.2 gives appropriate adjustment factors for the number of cases according to differing numbers of controls per case. For $c = 3$ the adjustment factor is 2/3. This means we would need $180 \times 2/3$, that is 120 cases, and three times as many, namely 360, controls. Thus although the requirement for the number of cases has considerably decreased, the total sample size has increased from 360 to 540.

CHAPTER 27

Use of Computers

Introduction

The past decade has seen a revolution in the accessibility of computer technology. Fifteen years ago few people even owned their own calculator, and the majority of hand-held calculators were rudimentary in performance, doing little more than basic arithmetic. Computers were mostly large machines requiring specially air-conditioned environments and several people to operate them. Their use was generally restricted to computer analysts and programmers. The advent of the microcomputer has changed all that. For relatively little cost, it is now possible to purchase one's own self-contained system that will fit on a desk-top and satisfy the majority of computing needs, and to acquire (even with no previous computer experience or background) fundamental computing skills in a relatively short time.

For all but the very smallest of studies, the use of a computer has many advantages. It is computationally faster and more accurate than doing the analyses by hand. Large data sets can be handled, and more complex analyses are possible. It is also easy to repeat an analysis with changes, for example to analyse males and females both separately and together. There are, however, a few warnings to be heeded. The use of a computer usually involves extra time in preparing data and programs. It is essential to check all procedures on a small subset of data and to validate the results by hand. Otherwise disastrous errors can occur. Finally, it is too easy to get carried away doing lots and lots of different analyses without really thinking about them.

We will now briefly describe the basic facilities needed for any computer system, and define common jargon. Since computer technology is moving so fast, no attempt will be made to make any definite recommendations about the type of equipment needed, nor will the list be comprehensive. An up-to-date specialist book or computer buyer's guide is recommended for more detail.

Computer hardware

Computer equipment is called **hardware**. A microcomputer will typically consist of a keyboard, a monitor (alternatively called a screen or visual display unit, VDU), a processor with memory (RAM = random access memory), and disk drives. It will usually have a printer attached.

A **mainframe** computer is a considerably more powerful processor, which has a time-sharing system dealing with several users at once. It has a more sophisticated operating system and a greater storage capacity. Data may be stored on hard disks for easy and quick access during analysis or on magnetic tape for more permanent storage of large volumes. The capacity of a magnetic tape depends on its length, density, and format. For example, a tape of 2400 feet written with a density of 1600 b.p.i. (bits per inch) could hold about 30 million characters of information. If this consisted of fairly long questionnaires, with say 120 variables, totalling 300 digits, the tape would hold about 100 000 questionnaires.

Disk drives

There are two types of **disk drives**, floppy and hard. A **floppy disk drive** can receive floppy disks (or diskettes), of varying sizes (for example, $3\frac{1}{2}''$, $5\frac{1}{4}''$ or 8″), depending on the particular machine. The capacity of a disk (and of the internal memory) is defined in terms of **bytes**, where one byte is the amount of space required to store one character. The capacity of a disk depends on the format the system uses for arranging data on the disk, whether information is stored in single or double density, and whether the disk drive can read one or both sides (single/double-sided). The letter 'k' is used to denote 1000, and mega means million. Thus a floppy disk with a capacity of 700 k can hold 7000 characters.

A **hard disk** usually comes in a fixed unit form, residing within the computer. It has a large capacity, for example 10 or 20 megabytes, and very fast reading and writing access.

Organization of data

Data are stored in **files**, which are listed in the **directory** of a disk. A file consists of **records**. There may be just one, or several, record(s) per individual, for example corresponding to different pages of the questionnaire. Files may be of either sequential or random access structure. In a **sequential file**, records are written or read in order. For example, to access the information relating to person number 10, it would first be necessary to read the information for persons 1–9. A **random access file**, on the other hand, is structured so that its records are identified and can be accessed by their numbers. It is possible to go straight to the position of record 10 to read (or write) the information for person number 10.

Records are written in either fixed or free format. In **fixed format** the data are arranged as a string of numbers (or characters), and a particular variable will always occupy the same column positions within the record. Numbers are right-justified. For example, if two positions have been allocated for age, then an age of 9 years would be stored as 09, or blank 9, but not as 9 blank. Decimal points are often not explicitly stored; their position is deduced from the column numbers. In **free format**, variables are simply arranged in order along the record, separated by commas or spaces. No attempt is made to make sure they line up from record to record. Decimal points must be entered. An example contrasting the two formats is given in Table 27.1.

Table 27.1 A comparison of fixed and free format for storing data.

ID	Age	Parity	Weight gain (kg)	Birth weight (g)
1	21	1	11.5	3520
2	18	0	9.5	2950
3	25	1	10.6	3380
4	31	3	14.1	3860
5	23	0	9.9	3200

Fixed format	*Free format*
12111153520	1, 21, 1, 11, 11.5, 3520
2180 952950	2, 18, 0, 9.5, 2950
32511063380	3, 25, 1, 10.6, 3380
43131413860	4, 31, 3, 14.1, 3860
5230 993200	5, 23, 0, 9.9, 3200

Finally, data are stored either directly as characters (**ascii** format) or first translated into machine form as a series of 0's and 1's (**binary** format). The format used will depend on how the file was created. Many software packages employ the binary format for any data handling and manipulation within the package, but then reproduce the file in ascii format if it is used with another package, or transferred to a different machine.

Back-up copies

It is essential to have at least three copies of any data file. Both disks and magnetic tapes can develop faults or get damaged. It is preferable to keep at least one copy in a different physical location to safeguard against events such as fires, floods, or theft. Back-up copies should be made regularly. The importance of this cannot be stressed enough.

Furthermore, when being entered into a computer, data are often stored intermediately in the computer memory and only transferred to the disk when this memory becomes full. It is good practice to ensure explicitly that the data are transferred at regular intervals, say every half an hour, to minimize the amount of data lost and time wasted if the computer malfunctions for some reason. Loss of power or a system failure due to a mistake, like trying to write more data to the disk than there is room for, or accidentally pressing a wrong combination of keys, will result in loss of memory and may even cause damage to the disk(s).

Computer software

No computer can operate without **software**. At the lowest level is the **operating system**, which consists of the commands needed to operate the computer, such as COPY a file, TYPE a file, RUN a program, list the DIRectory of a disk. Next comes a **program**, which is a set of instructions designed to do a task, for example to compare a child's weight with the median weight for age given in growth standards, and to express the observed weight as a percentage of the standard. A program is written in a **language**, such as Basic, Fortran, C or Pascal. The program is then translated into computer instructions by a **compiler**. Finally, a collection of programs with general applicability is called a **package**.

Packages of particular interest to us are of three types, database, statistical, and word-processing. A **database package** is recommended for data entry and general data organization, such as sorting and selection of subset of records. Most will reproduce the questionnaire on the screen and display the names of the variables being entered. A **cursor** will indicate the current position, and a bell will often sound when a complete questionnaire has been entered. Note that some packages have a fairly low restriction on the total number of variables that can be entered per individual, but that this can be overcome by combining variables and entering, for example, all anthropometric variables as one long variable.

Many database programs will also carry out tabulations and calculate basic statistics. In general, however, a specialized **statistical package** is recommended for data manipulation and analysis. A **word-processing package** is useful not only for report writing but also for program development, and for designing questionnaires. Linked to a database package, it may be possible in a follow-up study to use it to generate questionnaires which are partially completed with, for example, the individual's name, ID, address, and updated age, thus avoiding unnecessary manual copying from one survey to the next.

It is rare, however, that all requirements of a study can be satisfied by packages. There is usually a need to write a few small programs as well.

APPENDIX

Statistical Tables

Table A1 Areas in tail of the standard normal distribution.

Adapted from Table 3 of White *et al.* (1979) with permission of the authors and publishers.

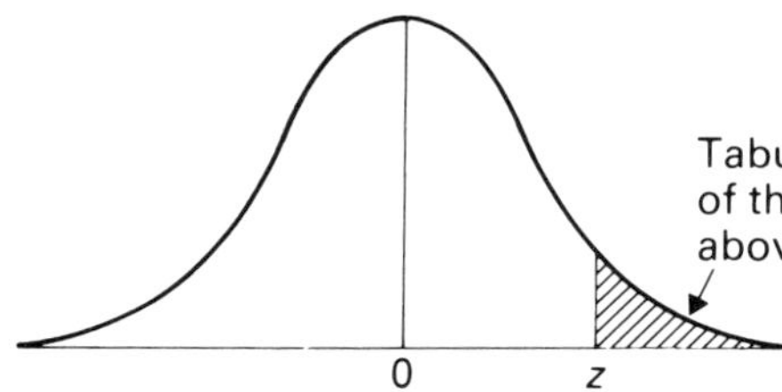

	Second decimal place of z									
z	0.00	0.01	0.02	0.03	0.04	0.05	0.06	0.07	0.08	0.09
0.0	0.5000	0.4960	0.4920	0.4880	0.4840	0.4801	0.4761	0.4721	0.4681	0.4641
0.1	0.4602	0.4562	0.4522	0.4483	0.4443	0.4404	0.4364	0.4325	0.4286	0.4247
0.2	0.4207	0.4168	0.4129	0.4090	0.4052	0.4013	0.3974	0.3936	0.3897	0.3859
0.3	0.3821	0.3783	0.3745	0.3707	0.3669	0.3632	0.3594	0.3557	0.3520	0.3483
0.4	0.3446	0.3409	0.3372	0.3336	0.3300	0.3264	0.3228	0.3192	0.3156	0.3121
0.5	0.3085	0.3050	0.3015	0.2981	0.2946	0.2912	0.2877	0.2843	0.2810	0.2776
0.6	0.2743	0.2709	0.2676	0.2643	0.2611	0.2578	0.2546	0.2514	0.2483	0.2451
0.7	0.2420	0.2389	0.2358	0.2327	0.2296	0.2266	0.2236	0.2206	0.2177	0.2148
0.8	0.2119	0.2090	0.2061	0.2033	0.2005	0.1977	0.1949	0.1922	0.1894	0.1867
0.9	0.1841	0.1814	0.1788	0.1762	0.1736	0.1711	0.1685	0.1660	0.1635	0.1611
1.0	0.1587	0.1562	0.1539	0.1515	0.1492	0.1469	0.1446	0.1423	0.1401	0.1379
1.1	0.1357	0.1335	0.1314	0.1292	0.1271	0.1251	0.1230	0.1210	0.1190	0.1170
1.2	0.1151	0.1131	0.1112	0.1093	0.1075	0.1056	0.1038	0.1020	0.1003	0.0985
1.3	0.0968	0.0951	0.0934	0.0918	0.0901	0.0885	0.0869	0.0853	0.0838	0.0823

1.6	0.0548	0.0537	0.0526	0.0516	0.0505	0.0495	0.0485	0.0475	0.0465	0.0455
1.7	0.0446	0.0436	0.0427	0.0418	0.0409	0.0401	0.0392	0.0384	0.0375	0.0367
1.8	0.0359	0.0351	0.0344	0.0336	0.0329	0.0322	0.0314	0.0307	0.0301	0.0294
1.9	0.0287	0.0281	0.0274	0.0268	0.0262	0.0256	0.0250	0.0244	0.0239	0.0233
2.0	0.02275	0.02222	0.02169	0.02118	0.02068	0.02018	0.01970	0.01923	0.01876	0.01831
2.1	0.01786	0.01743	0.01700	0.01659	0.01618	0.01578	0.01539	0.01500	0.01463	0.01426
2.2	0.01390	0.01355	0.01321	0.01287	0.01255	0.01222	0.01191	0.01160	0.01130	0.01101
2.3	0.01072	0.01044	0.01017	0.00990	0.00964	0.00939	0.00914	0.00889	0.00866	0.00842
2.4	0.00820	0.00798	0.00776	0.00755	0.00734	0.00714	0.00695	0.00676	0.00657	0.00639
2.5	0.00621	0.00604	0.00587	0.00570	0.00554	0.00539	0.00523	0.00508	0.00494	0.00480
2.6	0.00466	0.00453	0.00440	0.00427	0.00415	0.00402	0.00391	0.00379	0.00368	0.00357
2.7	0.00347	0.00336	0.00326	0.00317	0.00307	0.00298	0.00289	0.00280	0.00272	0.00264
2.8	0.00256	0.00248	0.00240	0.00233	0.00226	0.00219	0.00212	0.00205	0.00199	0.00193
2.9	0.00187	0.00181	0.00175	0.00169	0.00164	0.00159	0.00154	0.00149	0.00144	0.00139
3.0	0.00135	0.00131	0.00126	0.00122	0.00118	0.00114	0.00111	0.00107	0.00104	0.00100
3.1	0.00097	0.00094	0.00090	0.00087	0.00084	0.00082	0.00079	0.00076	0.00074	0.00071
3.2	0.00069	0.00066	0.00064	0.00062	0.00060	0.00058	0.00056	0.00054	0.00052	0.00050
3.3	0.00048	0.00047	0.00045	0.00043	0.00042	0.00040	0.00039	0.00038	0.00036	0.00035
3.4	0.00034	0.00032	0.00031	0.00030	0.00029	0.00028	0.00027	0.00026	0.00025	0.00024
3.5	0.00023	0.00022	0.00022	0.00021	0.00020	0.00019	0.00019	0.00018	0.00017	0.00017
3.6	0.00016	0.00015	0.00015	0.00014	0.00014	0.00013	0.00013	0.00012	0.00012	0.00011
3.7	0.00011	0.00010	0.00010	0.00010	0.00009	0.00009	0.00008	0.00008	0.00008	0.00008
3.8	0.00007	0.00007	0.00007	0.00006	0.00006	0.00006	0.00006	0.00005	0.00005	0.00005
3.9	0.00005	0.00005	0.00004	0.00004	0.00004	0.00004	0.00004	0.00004	0.00003	0.00003

Table A2 Percentage points of the standard normal distribution.

	Percentage points	
P value	One-sided	Two-sided
0.5	0.00	0.67
0.4	0.25	0.84
0.3	0.52	1.04
0.2	0.84	1.28
0.1	1.28	1.64
0.05	1.64	1.96
0.02	2.05	2.33
0.01	2.33	2.58
0.005	2.58	2.81
0.002	2.88	3.09
0.001	3.09	3.29
0.0001	3.72	3.89

Table A3 Percentage points of the *t* distribution.

Adapted from Table 7 of White *et al.* (1979) with permission of authors and publishers.

	One-sided *P* value								
	0.25	0.1	0.05	0.025	0.01	0.005	0.0025	0.001	0.0005
	Two-sided *P* value								
d.f.	0.5	0.2	0.1	0.05	0.02	0.01	0.005	0.002	0.001
1	1.00	3.08	6.31	12.71	31.82	63.66	127.32	318.31	636.62
2	0.82	1.89	2.92	4.30	6.96	9.92	14.09	22.33	31.60
3	0.76	1.64	2.35	3.18	4.54	5.84	7.45	10.21	12.92
4	0.74	1.53	2.13	2.78	3.75	4.60	5.60	7.17	8.61
5	0.73	1.48	2.02	2.57	3.36	4.03	4.77	5.89	6.87
6	0.72	1.44	1.94	2.45	3.14	3.71	4.32	5.21	5.96
7	0.71	1.42	1.90	2.36	3.00	3.50	4.03	4.78	5.41
8	0.71	1.40	1.86	2.31	2.90	3.36	3.83	4.50	5.04
9	0.70	1.38	1.83	2.26	2.82	3.25	3.69	4.30	4.78
10	0.70	1.37	1.81	2.23	2.76	3.17	3.58	4.14	4.59
11	0.70	1.36	1.80	2.20	2.72	3.11	3.50	4.02	4.44
12	0.70	1.36	1.78	2.18	2.68	3.06	3.43	3.93	4.32
13	0.69	1.35	1.77	2.16	2.65	3.01	3.37	3.85	4.22
14	0.69	1.34	1.76	2.14	2.62	2.98	3.33	3.79	4.14
15	0.69	1.34	1.75	2.13	2.60	2.95	3.29	3.73	4.07
16	0.69	1.34	1.75	2.12	2.58	2.92	3.25	3.69	4.02
17	0.69	1.33	1.74	2.11	2.57	2.90	3.22	3.65	3.96
18	0.69	1.33	1.73	2.10	2.55	2.88	3.20	3.61	3.92
19	0.69	1.33	1.73	2.09	2.54	2.86	3.17	3.58	3.88
20	0.69	1.32	1.72	2.09	2.53	2.84	3.15	3.55	3.85
21	0.69	1.32	1.72	2.08	2.52	2.83	3.14	3.53	3.82
22	0.69	1.32	1.72	2.07	2.51	2.82	3.12	3.50	3.79
23	0.68	1.32	1.71	2.07	2.50	2.81	3.10	3.48	3.77
24	0.68	1.32	1.71	2.06	2.49	2.80	3.09	3.47	3.74
25	0.68	1.32	1.71	2.06	2.48	2.79	3.08	3.45	3.72
26	0.68	1.32	1.71	2.06	2.48	2.78	3.07	3.44	3.71
27	0.68	1.31	1.70	2.05	2.47	2.77	3.06	3.42	3.69
28	0.68	1.31	1.70	2.05	2.47	2.76	3.05	3.41	3.67
29	0.68	1.31	1.70	2.04	2.46	2.76	3.04	3.40	3.66
30	0.68	1.31	1.70	2.04	2.46	2.75	3.03	3.38	3.65
40	0.68	1.30	1.68	2.02	2.42	2.70	2.97	3.31	3.55
60	0.68	1.30	1.67	2.00	2.39	2.66	2.92	3.23	3.46
120	0.68	1.29	1.66	1.98	2.36	2.62	2.86	3.16	3.37
∞	0.67	1.28	1.65	1.96	2.33	2.58	2.81	3.09	3.29

Table A4 Percentage points of the F distribution.

Adapted from Table 4 of Armitage (1971) and Table 18 of Pearson & Hartley (1966) with permission of the authors and publishers and the Biometrika Trustees.

The table gives a one-sided significance test for the comparison of two variances, as appropriate for use in analysis of variance. A two-sided test may be obtained by doubling the P values.

$d.f._1$ = d.f. for numerator; $d.f._2$ = d.f. for denominator

		$d.f._1$														
$d.f._2$	P value	1	2	3	4	5	6	7	8	9	10	20	40	60	120	∞
1	0.05	161	200	216	225	230	234	237	239	241	242	248	251	252	253	254
	0.025	648	800	864	900	922	937	948	957	963	969	993	1006	1010	1014	1018
	0.01	4052	5000	5403	5625	5764	5859	5928	5981	6022	6056	6209	6287	6313	6339	6366
	0.005	16211	20000	21615	22500	23056	23437	23715	23925	24091	24224	24836	25148	25253	25359	25465
	0.001	405300	500000	540400	562500	576400	585900	592900	598100	602300	605600	620900	628700	631300	634000	636600
2	0.05	18.51	19.00	19.16	19.25	19.30	19.33	19.35	19.37	19.38	19.40	19.45	19.47	19.48	19.49	19.50
	0.025	38.51	39.00	39.17	39.25	39.30	39.33	39.36	39.37	39.39	39.40	39.45	39.47	39.48	39.49	39.50
	0.01	98.50	99.00	99.17	99.25	99.30	99.33	99.36	99.37	99.39	99.40	99.45	99.47	99.48	99.49	99.50
	0.005	198.5	199.0	199.2	199.2	199.3	199.3	199.4	199.4	199.4	199.4	199.4	199.5	199.5	199.5	199.5
	0.001	998.5	999.0	999.2	999.2	999.3	999.3	999.4	999.4	999.4	999.4	999.4	999.5	999.5	999.5	999.5
3	0.05	10.13	9.55	9.28	9.12	9.01	8.94	8.89	8.85	8.81	8.79	8.66	8.59	8.57	8.55	8.53
	0.025	17.44	16.04	15.44	15.10	14.88	14.73	14.62	14.54	14.47	14.42	14.17	14.04	13.99	13.95	13.90
	0.01	34.12	30.82	29.46	28.71	28.24	27.91	27.67	27.49	27.35	27.23	26.69	26.41	26.32	26.22	26.13
	0.005	55.55	49.80	47.47	46.19	45.39	44.84	44.43	44.13	43.88	43.69	42.78	42.31	42.15	41.99	41.83
	0.001	167.0	148.5	141.1	137.1	134.6	132.8	131.6	130.6	129.9	129.2	126.4	125.0	124.5	124.0	123.5
4	0.05	7.71	6.94	6.59	6.39	6.26	6.16	6.09	6.04	6.00	5.96	5.80	5.72	5.69	5.66	5.63
	0.025	12.22	10.65	9.98	9.60	9.36	9.20	9.07	8.98	8.90	8.84	8.56	8.41	8.36	8.31	8.26
	0.01	21.20	18.00	16.69	15.98	15.52	15.21	14.98	14.80	14.66	14.55	14.02	13.75	13.65	13.56	13.46
	0.005	31.33	26.28	24.26	23.15	22.46	21.97	21.62	21.35	21.14	20.97	20.17	19.75	19.61	19.47	19.32
	0.001	74.14	61.25	56.18	53.44	51.71	50.53	49.66	49.00	48.47	48.05	46.10	45.09	44.75	44.40	44.05

5	0.05	6.61	5.79	5.41	5.19	5.05	4.95	4.88	4.82	4.77	4.74	4.56	4.46	4.43	4.40	4.36
	0.025	10·01	8.43	7.76	7.39	7.15	6.98	6.85	6.76	6.68	6.62	6.33	6.18	6.12	6.07	6.02
	0.01	16.26	13.27	12.06	11.39	10.97	10.67	10.46	10.29	10.16	10.05	9.55	9.29	9.20	9.11	9.02
	0.005	22.78	18.31	16.53	15.56	14.94	14.51	14.20	13.96	13.77	13.62	12.90	12.53	12.40	12.27	12.14
	0.001	47.18	37.12	33.20	31.09	29.75	28.84	28.16	27.64	27.24	26.92	25.39	24.60	24.33	24.06	23.79
6	0.05	5.99	5.14	4.76	4.53	4.39	4.28	4.21	4.15	4.10	4.06	3.87	3.77	3.74	3.70	3.67
	0.025	8.81	7.26	6.60	6.23	5.99	5.82	5.70	5.60	5.52	5.46	5.17	5.01	4.96	4.90	4.85
	0.01	13.75	10.92	9.78	9.15	8.75	8.47	8.26	8.10	7.98	7.87	7.40	7.14	7.06	6.97	6.88
	0.005	18.63	14.54	12.92	12.03	11.46	11.07	10.79	10.57	10.39	10.25	9.59	9.24	9.12	9.00	8.88
	0.001	35.51	27.00	23.70	21.92	20.81	20.03	19.46	19.03	18.69	18.41	17.12	16.44	16.21	15.99	15.75
7	0.05	5.59	4.74	4.35	4.12	3.97	3.87	3.79	3.73	3.68	3.64	3.44	3.34	3.30	3.27	3.23
	0.025	8.07	6.54	5.89	5.52	5.29	5.12	4.99	4.90	4.82	4.76	4.47	4.31	4.25	4.20	4.14
	0.01	12.25	9.55	8.45	7.85	7.46	7.19	6.99	6.84	6.72	6.62	6.16	5.91	5.82	5.74	5.65
	0.005	16.24	12.40	10.88	10.05	9.52	9.16	8.89	8.68	8.51	8.38	7.75	7.42	7.31	7.19	7.08
	0.001	29.25	21.69	18.77	17.19	16.21	15.52	15.02	14.63	14.33	14.08	12.93	12.33	12.12	11.91	11.70
8	0.05	5.32	4.46	4.07	3.84	3.69	3.58	3.50	3.44	3.39	3.35	3.15	3.04	3.01	2.97	2.93
	0.025	7.57	6.06	5.42	5.05	4.82	4.65	4.53	4.43	4.36	4.30	4.00	3.84	3.78	3.73	3.67
	0.01	11.26	8.65	7.59	7.01	6.63	6.37	6.18	6.03	5.91	5.81	5.36	5.12	5.03	4.95	4.86
	0.005	14.69	11.04	9.60	8.81	8.30	7.95	7.69	7.50	7.34	7.21	6.61	6.29	6.18	6.06	5.95
	0.001	25.42	18.49	15.83	14.39	13.49	12.86	12.40	12.04	11.77	11.54	10.48	9.92	9.73	9.53	9.33
9	0.05	5.12	4.26	3.86	3.63	3.48	3.37	3.29	3.23	3.18	3.14	2.94	2.83	2.79	2.75	2.71
	0.025	7.21	5.71	5.08	4.72	4.48	4.32	4.20	4.10	4.03	3.96	3.67	3.51	3.45	3.39	3.33
	0.01	10.56	8.02	6.99	6.42	6.06	5.80	5.61	5.47	5.35	5.26	4.81	4.57	4.48	4.40	4.31
	0.005	13.61	10.11	8.72	7.96	7.47	7.13	6.88	6.69	6.54	6.42	5.83	5.52	5.41	5.30	5.19
	0.001	22.86	16.39	13.90	12.56	11.71	11.13	10.70	10.37	10.11	9.89	8.90	8.37	8.19	8.00	7.81
10	0.05	4.96	4.10	3.71	3.48	3.33	3.22	3.14	3.07	3.02	2.98	2.77	2.66	2.62	2.58	2.54
	0.025	6.94	5.46	4.83	4.47	4.24	4.07	3.95	3.85	3.78	3.72	3.42	3.26	3.20	3.14	3.08
	0.01	10.04	7.56	6.55	5.99	5.64	5.39	5.20	5.06	4.94	4.85	4.41	4.17	4.08	4.00	3.91
	0.005	12.83	9.43	8.08	7.34	6.87	6.54	6.30	6.12	5.97	5.85	5.27	4.97	4.86	4.75	4.64
	0.001	21.04	14.91	12.55	11.28	10.48	9.92	9.52	9.20	8.96	8.75	7.80	7.30	7.12	6.94	6.76

Table A4 Percentage points of the F distribution *(continued)*

		d.f.$_1$														
d.f.$_2$	P value	1	2	3	4	5	6	7	8	9	10	20	40	60	120	∞
12	0.05	4.75	3.89	3.49	3.26	3.11	3.00	2.91	2.85	2.80	2.75	2.54	2.43	2.38	2.34	2.30
	0.025	6.55	5.10	4.47	4.12	3.89	3.73	3.61	3.51	3.44	3.37	3.07	2.91	2.85	2.79	2.72
	0.01	9.33	6.93	5.95	5.41	5.06	4.82	4.64	4.50	4.39	4.30	3.86	3.62	3.54	3.45	3.36
	0.005	11.75	8.51	7.23	6.52	6.07	5.76	5.52	5.35	5.20	5.09	4.53	4.23	4.12	4.01	3.90
	0.001	18.64	12.97	10.80	9.63	8.89	8.38	8.00	7.71	7.48	7.29	6.40	5.93	5.76	5.59	5.42
14	0.05	4.60	3.74	3.34	3.11	2.96	2.85	2.76	2.70	2.65	2.60	2.39	2.27	2.22	2.18	2.13
	0.025	6.30	4.86	4.24	3.89	3.66	3.50	3.38	3.29	3.21	3.15	2.84	2.67	2.61	2.55	2.49
	0.01	8.86	6.51	5.56	5.04	4.69	4.46	4.28	4.14	4.03	3.94	3.51	3.27	3.18	3.09	3.00
	0.005	11.06	7.92	6.68	6.00	5.56	5.26	5.03	4.86	4.72	4.60	4.06	3.76	3.66	3.55	3.44
	0.001	17.14	11.78	9.73	8.62	7.92	7.43	7.08	6.80	6.58	6.40	5.56	5.10	4.94	4.77	4.60
16	0.05	4.49	3.63	3.24	3.01	2.85	2.74	2.66	2.59	2.54	2.49	2.28	2.15	2.11	2.06	2.01
	0.025	6.12	4.69	4.08	3.73	3.50	3.34	3.22	3.12	3.05	2.99	2.68	2.51	2.45	2.38	2.32
	0.01	8.53	6.23	5.29	4.77	4.44	4.20	4.03	3.89	3.78	3.69	3.26	3.02	2.93	2.84	2.75
	0.005	10.58	7.51	6.30	5.64	5.21	4.91	4.69	4.52	4.38	4.27	3.73	3.44	3.33	3.22	3.11
	0.001	16.12	10.97	9.00	7.94	7.27	6.81	6.46	6.19	5.98	5.81	4.99	4.54	4.39	4.23	4.06
18	0.05	4.41	3.55	3.16	2.93	2.77	2.66	2.58	2.51	2.46	2.41	2.19	2.06	2.02	1.97	1.92
	0.025	5.98	4.56	3.95	3.61	3.38	3.22	3.10	3.01	2.93	2.87	2.56	2.38	2.32	2.26	2.19
	0.01	8.29	6.01	5.09	4.58	4.25	4.01	3.84	3.71	3.60	3.51	3.08	2.84	2.75	2.66	2.57
	0.005	10.22	7.21	6.03	5.37	4.96	4.66	4.44	4.28	4.14	4.03	3.50	3.20	3.10	2.99	2.87
	0.001	15.38	10.39	8.49	7.46	6.81	6.35	6.02	5.76	5.56	5.39	4.59	4.15	4.00	3.84	3.67
20	0.05	4.35	3.49	3.10	2.87	2.71	2.60	2.51	2.45	2.39	2.35	2.12	1.99	1.95	1.90	1.84
	0.025	5.87	4.46	3.86	3.51	3.29	3.13	3.01	2.91	2.84	2.77	2.46	2.29	2.22	2.16	2.09
	0.01	8.10	5.85	4.94	4.43	4.10	3.87	3.70	3.56	3.46	3.37	2.94	2.69	2.61	2.52	2.42
	0.005	9.94	6.99	5.82	5.17	4.76	4.47	4.26	4.09	3.96	3.85	3.82	3.02	2.92	2.81	2.69
	0.001	14.82	9.95	8.10	7.10	6.46	6.02	5.69	5.44	5.24	5.08	4.29	3.86	3.70	3.54	3.38

25	0.05	4.24	3.39	2.99	2.76	2.60	2.49	2.40	2.34	2.28	2.24	2.01	1.87	1.82	1.77	1.71
	0.025	5.69	4.29	3.69	3.35	3.13	2.97	2.85	2.75	2.68	2.61	2.30	2.12	2.05	1.98	1.91
	0.01	7.77	5.57	4.68	4.18	3.85	3.63	3.46	3.32	3.22	3.13	2.70	2.45	2.36	2.27	2.17
	0.005	9.48	6.60	5.46	4.84	4.43	4.15	3.94	3.78	3.64	3.54	3.01	2.72	2.61	2.50	2.38
	0.001	13.88	9.22	7.45	6.49	5.88	5.46	5.15	4.91	4.71	4.56	3.79	3.37	3.22	3.06	2.89
30	0.05	4.17	3.32	2.92	2.69	2.53	2.42	2.33	2.27	2.21	2.16	1.93	1.79	1.74	1.68	1.62
	0.025	5.57	4.18	3.59	3.25	3.03	2.87	2.75	2.65	2.57	2.51	2.20	2.01	1.94	1.87	1.79
	0.01	7.56	5.39	4.51	4.02	3.70	3.47	3.30	3.17	3.07	2.98	2.55	2.30	2.21	2.11	2.01
	0.005	9.18	6.35	5.24	4.62	4.23	3.95	3.74	3.58	3.45	3.34	2.82	2.52	2.42	2.30	2.18
	0.001	13.29	8.77	7.05	6.12	5.53	5.12	4.82	4.58	4.39	4.24	3.49	3.07	2.92	2.76	2.59
40	0.05	4.08	3.23	2.84	2.61	2.45	2.34	2.25	2.18	2.12	2.08	1.84	1.69	1.64	1.58	1.51
	0.025	5.42	4.05	3.46	3.13	2.90	2.74	2.62	2.53	2.45	2.39	2.07	1.88	1.80	1.72	1.64
	0.01	7.31	5.18	4.31	3.83	3.51	3.29	3.12	2.99	2.89	2.80	2.37	2.11	2.02	1.92	1.80
	0.005	8.83	6.07	4.98	4.37	3.99	3.71	3.51	3.35	3.22	3.12	2.60	2.30	2.18	2.06	1.93
	0.001	12.61	8.25	6.60	5.70	5.13	4.73	4.44	4.21	4.02	3.87	3.15	2.73	2.57	2.41	2.23
60	0.05	4.00	3.15	2.76	2.53	2.37	2.25	2.17	2.10	2.04	1.99	1.75	1.59	1.53	1.47	1.39
	0.025	5.29	3.93	3.34	3.01	2.79	2.63	2.51	2.41	2.33	2.27	1.94	1.74	1.67	1.58	1.48
	0.01	7.08	4.98	4.13	3.65	3.34	3.12	2.95	2.82	2.72	2.63	2.20	1.94	1.84	1.73	1.60
	0.005	8.49	5.79	4.73	4.14	3.76	3.49	3.29	3.13	3.01	2.90	2.39	2.08	1.96	1.83	1.69
	0.001	11.97	7.76	6.17	5.31	4.76	4.37	4.09	3.87	3.69	3.54	2.83	2.41	2.25	2.08	1.89
120	0.05	3.92	3.07	2.68	2.45	2.29	2.17	2.09	2.02	1.96	1.91	1.66	1.50	1.43	1.35	1.25
	0.025	5.15	3.80	3.23	2.89	2.67	2.52	2.39	2.30	2.22	2.16	1.82	1.61	1.53	1.43	1.31
	0.01	6.85	4.79	3.95	3.48	3.17	2.96	2.79	2.66	2.56	2.47	2.03	1.76	1.66	1.53	1.38
	0.005	8.18	5.54	4.50	3.92	3.55	3.28	3.09	2.93	2.81	2.71	2.19	1.87	1.75	1.61	1.43
	0.001	11.38	7.32	5.79	4.95	4.42	4.04	3.77	3.55	3.38	3.24	2.53	2.11	1.95	1.76	1.54
∞	0.05	3.84	3.00	2.60	2.37	2.21	2.10	2.01	1.94	1.88	1.83	1.57	1.39	1.32	1.22	1.00
	0.025	5.02	3.69	3.12	2.79	2.57	2.41	2.29	2.19	2.11	2.05	1.71	1.48	1.39	1.27	1.00
	0.01	6.63	4.61	3.78	3.32	3.02	2.80	2.64	2.51	2.41	2.32	1.88	1.59	1.47	1.32	1.00
	0.005	7.88	5.30	4.28	3.72	3.35	3.09	2.90	2.74	2.62	2.52	2.00	1.67	1.53	1.36	1.00
	0.001	10.83	6.91	5.42	4.62	4.10	3.74	3.47	3.27	3.10	2.96	2.27	1.84	1.66	1.45	1.00

Table A5 Percentage points of the χ^2 distribution.

Adapted from Table 8 of White *et al.* (1979) with permission of the authors and publishers.

d.f. = 1. In the comparison of two proportions (2×2 χ^2 or Mantel–Haenszel χ^2 test) or in the assessment of a trend, the percentage points give a two-sided test. A one-sided test may be obtained by halving the *P* values. (Concepts of one- and two-sidedness do not apply to larger degrees of freedom, as these relate to tests of multiple comparisons.)

	P value							
d.f.	0.5	0.25	0.1	0.05	0.025	0.01	0.005	0.001
1	0.45	1.32	2.71	3.84	5.02	6.63	7.88	10.83
2	1.39	2.77	4.61	5.99	7.38	9.21	10.60	13.82
3	2.37	4.11	6.25	7.81	9.35	11.34	12.84	16.27
4	3.36	5.39	7.78	9.49	11.14	13.28	14.86	18.47
5	4.35	6.63	9.24	11.07	12.83	15.09	16.75	20.52
6	5.35	7.84	10.64	12.59	14.45	16.81	18.55	22.46
7	6.35	9.04	12.02	14.07	16.01	18.48	20.28	24.32
8	7.34	10.22	13.36	15.51	17.53	20.09	21.96	26.13
9	8.34	11.39	14.68	16.92	19.02	21.67	23.59	27.88
10	9.34	12.55	15.99	18.31	20.48	23.21	25.19	29.59
11	10.34	13.70	17.28	19.68	21.92	24.73	26.76	31.26
12	11.34	14.85	18.55	21.03	23.34	26.22	28.30	32.91
13	12.34	15.98	19.81	22.36	24.74	27.69	29.82	34.53
14	13.34	17.12	21.06	23.68	26.12	29.14	31.32	36.12
15	14.34	18.25	22.31	25.00	27.49	30.58	32.80	37.70
16	15.34	19.37	23.54	26.30	28.85	32.00	34.27	39.25
17	16.34	20.49	24.77	27.59	30.19	33.41	35.72	40.79
18	17.34	21.60	25.99	28.87	31.53	34.81	37.16	42.31
19	18.34	22.72	27.20	30.14	32.85	36.19	38.58	43.82
20	19.34	23.83	28.41	31.41	34.17	37.57	40.00	45.32
21	20.34	24.93	29.62	32.67	35.48	38.93	41.40	46.80
22	21.34	26.04	30.81	33.92	36.78	40.29	42.80	48.27
23	22.34	27.14	32.01	35.17	38.08	41.64	44.18	49.73
24	23.34	28.24	33.20	36.42	39.36	42.98	45.56	51.18
25	24.34	29.34	34.38	37.65	40.65	44.31	46.93	52.62
26	25.34	30.43	35.56	38.89	41.92	45.64	48.29	54.05
27	26.34	31.53	36.74	40.11	43.19	46.96	49.64	55.48
28	27.34	32.62	37.92	41.34	44.46	48.28	50.99	56.89
29	28.34	33.71	39.09	42.56	45.72	49.59	52.34	58.30
30	29.34	34.80	40.26	43.77	46.98	50.89	53.67	59.70
40	39.34	45.62	51.81	55.76	59.34	63.69	66.77	73.40
50	49.33	56.33	63.17	67.50	71.42	76.15	79.49	86.66
60	59.33	66.98	74.40	79.08	83.30	88.38	91.95	99.61
70	69.33	77.58	85.53	90.53	95.02	100.43	104.22	112.32
80	79.33	88.13	96.58	101.88	106.63	112.33	116.32	124.84
90	89.33	98.65	107.57	113.15	118.14	124.12	128.30	137.21
100	99.33	109.14	118.50	124.34	129.56	135.81	140.17	149.45

Table A6 Probits.

Adapted from Table 4 of Pearson & Hartley (1966) with permission of the Biometrika Trustees

Probit =	value of standard normal distribution corresponding to cumulative percentage	+5, optional: not included in this table

%	0.0	0.1	0.2	0.3	0.4	0.5	0.6	0.7	0.8	0.9
	Decimal place of %									
0	−∞	−3.09	−2.88	−2.75	−2.65	−2.58	−2.51	−2.46	−2.41	−2.37
1	−2.33	−2.29	−2.26	−2.23	−2.20	−2.17	−2.14	−2.12	−2.10	−2.07
2	−2.05	−2.03	−2.01	−2.00	−1.98	−1.96	−1.94	−1.93	−1.91	−1.90
3	−1.88	−1.87	−1.85	−1.84	−1.83	−1.81	−1.80	−1.79	−1.77	−1.76
4	−1.75	−1.74	−1.73	−1.72	−1.71	−1.70	−1.68	−1.67	−1.66	−1.65
5	−1.64	−1.64	−1.63	−1.62	−1.61	−1.60	−1.59	−1.58	−1.57	−1.56
6	−1.55	−1.55	−1.54	−1.53	−1.52	−1.51	−1.51	−1.50	−1.49	−1.48
7	−1.48	−1.47	−1.46	−1.45	−1.45	−1.44	−1.43	−1.43	−1.42	−1.41
8	−1.41	−1.40	−1.39	−1.39	−1.38	−1.37	−1.37	−1.36	−1.35	−1.35
9	−1.34	−1.33	−1.33	−1.32	−1.32	−1.31	−1.30	−1.30	−1.29	−1.29
10	−1.28	−1.28	−1.27	−1.26	−1.26	−1.25	−1.25	−1.24	−1.24	−1.23
11	−1.23	−1.22	−1.22	−1.21	−1.21	−1.20	−1.20	−1.19	−1.19	−1.18
12	−1.18	−1.17	−1.17	−1.16	−1.16	−1.15	−1.15	−1.14	−1.14	−1.13
13	−1.13	−1.12	−1.12	−1.11	−1.11	−1.10	−1.10	−1.09	−1.09	−1.08
14	−1.08	−1.08	−1.07	−1.07	−1.06	−1.06	−1.05	−1.05	−1.05	−1.04
15	−1.04	−1.03	−1.03	−1.02	−1.02	−1.02	−1.01	−1.01	−1.00	−1.00
16	−0.99	−0.99	−0.99	−0.98	−0.98	−0.97	−0.97	−0.97	−0.96	−0.96
17	−0.95	−0.95	−0.95	−0.94	−0.94	−0.93	−0.93	−0.93	−0.92	−0.92
18	−0.92	−0.91	−0.91	−0.90	−0.90	−0.90	−0.89	−0.89	−0.89	−0.88
19	−0·88	−0.87	−0.87	−0.87	−0.86	−0.86	−0.86	−0.85	−0.85	−0.85
20	−0·84	−0.84	−0.83	−0.83	−0.83	−0.82	−0.82	−0.82	−0.81	−0.81
21	−0.81	−0.80	−0.80	−0.80	−0.79	−0.79	−0.79	−0.78	−0.78	−0.78
22	−0.77	−0.77	−0.77	−0.76	−0.76	−0.76	−0.75	−0.75	−0.75	−0.74
23	−0.74	−0.74	−0.73	−0.73	−0.73	−0.72	−0.72	−0.72	−0.71	−0.71
24	−0·71	−0.70	−0.70	−0.70	−0.69	−0.69	−0.69	−0.68	−0.68	−0.68
25	−0.67	−0.67	−0.67	−0.67	−0.66	−0.66	−0.66	−0.65	−0.65	−0.65
26	−0.64	−0.64	−0.64	−0.63	−0.63	−0.63	−0.63	−0.62	−0.62	−0.62
27	−0.61	−0.61	−0.61	−0.60	−0.60	−0.60	−0.59	−0.59	−0.59	−0.59
28	−0.58	−0.58	−0.58	−0.57	−0.57	−0.57	−0.57	−0.56	−0.56	−0.56
29	−0.55	−0.55	−0.55	−0.54	−0.54	−0.54	−0.54	−0.53	−0.53	−0.53
30	−0.52	−0.52	−0.52	−0.52	−0.51	−0.51	−0.51	−0.50	−0.50	−0.50
31	−0.50	−0.49	−0.49	−0.49	−0.48	−0.48	−0.48	−0.48	−0.47	−0.47
32	−0.47	−0.46	−0.46	−0.46	−0.46	−0.45	−0.45	−0.45	−0.45	−0.44
33	−0.44	−0.44	−0.43	−0.43	−0.43	−0.43	−0.42	−0.42	−0.42	−0.42
34	−0.41	−0.41	−0.41	−0.40	−0.40	−0.40	−0.40	−0.39	−0.39	−0.39
35	−0.39	−0.38	−0.38	−0.38	−0.37	−0.37	−0.37	−0.37	−0.36	−0.36
36	−0.36	−0.36	−0.35	−0.35	−0.35	−0.35	−0.34	−0.34	−0.34	−0.33
37	−0.33	−0.33	−0.33	−0.32	−0.32	−0.32	−0.32	−0.31	−0.31	−0.31
38	−0.31	−0.30	−0.30	−0.30	−0.30	−0.29	−0.29	−0.29	−0.28	−0.28
39	−0.28	−0.28	−0.27	−0.27	−0.27	−0.27	−0.26	−0.26	−0.26	−0.26
40	−0.25	−0.25	−0.25	−0.25	−0.24	−0.24	−0.24	−0.24	−0.23	−0.23
41	−0.23	−0.23	−0.22	−0.22	−0.22	−0.21	−0.21	−0.21	−0.21	−0.20
42	−0.20	−0.20	−0.20	−0.19	−0.19	−0.19	−0.19	−0.18	−0.18	−0.18
43	−0.18	−0.17	−0.17	−0.17	−0.17	−0.16	−0.16	−0.16	−0.16	−0.15
44	−0.15	−0.15	−0.15	−0.14	−0.14	−0.14	−0.14	−0.13	−0.13	−0.13
45	−0.13	−0.12	−0.12	−0.12	−0.12	−0.11	−0.11	−0.11	−0.11	−0.10
46	−0.10	−0.10	−0.10	−0.09	−0.09	−0.09	−0.09	−0.08	−0.08	−0.08
47	−0.08	−0.07	−0.07	−0.07	−0.07	−0.06	−0.06	−0.06	−0.06	−0.05
48	−0.05	−0.05	−0.05	−0.04	−0.04	−0.04	−0.04	−0.03	−0.03	−0.03
49	−0.03	−0.02	−0.02	−0.02	−0.02	−0.01	−0.01	−0.01	−0.01	0.00

Table A6 Probits *continued*

	Decimal place of %									
%	0.0	0.1	0.2	0.3	0.4	0.5	0.6	0.7	0.8	0.9
50	0.00	0.00	0.01	0.01	0.01	0.01	0.02	0.02	0.02	0.02
51	0.03	0.03	0.03	0.03	0.04	0.04	0.04	0.04	0.05	0.05
52	0.05	0.05	0.06	0.06	0.06	0.06	0.07	0.07	0.07	0.07
53	0.08	0.08	0.08	0.08	0.09	0.09	0.09	0.09	0.10	0.10
54	0.10	0.10	0.11	0.11	0.11	0.11	0.12	0.12	0.12	0.12
55	0.13	0.13	0.13	0.13	0.14	0.14	0.14	0.14	0.15	0.15
56	0.15	0.15	0.16	0.16	0.16	0.16	0.17	0.17	0.17	0.17
57	0.18	0.18	0.18	0.18	0.19	0.19	0.19	0.19	0.20	0.20
58	0.20	0.20	0.21	0.21	0.21	0.21	0.22	0.22	0.22	0.23
59	0.23	0.23	0.23	0.24	0.24	0.24	0.24	0.25	0.25	0.25
60	0.25	0.26	0.26	0.26	0.26	0.27	0.27	0.27	0.27	0.28
61	0.28	0.28	0.28	0.29	0.29	0.29	0.30	0.30	0.30	0.30
62	0.31	0.31	0.31	0.31	0.32	0.32	0.32	0.32	0.33	0.33
63	0.33	0.33	0.34	0.34	0.34	0.35	0.35	0.35	0.35	0.36
64	0.36	0.36	0.36	0.37	0.37	0.37	0.37	0.38	0.38	0.38
65	0.39	0.39	0.39	0.39	0.40	0.40	0.40	0.40	0.41	0.41
66	0.41	0.42	0.42	0.42	0.42	0.43	0.43	0.43	0.43	0.44
67	0.44	0.44	0.45	0.45	0.45	0.45	0.46	0.46	0.46	0.46
68	0.47	0.47	0.47	0.48	0.48	0.48	0.48	0.49	0.49	0.49
69	0.50	0.50	0.50	0.50	0.51	0.51	0.51	0.52	0.52	0.52
70	0.52	0.53	0.53	0.53	0.54	0.54	0.54	0.54	0.55	0.55
71	0.55	0.56	0.56	0.56	0.57	0.57	0.57	0.57	0.58	0.58
72	0.58	0.59	0.59	0.59	0.59	0.60	0.60	0.60	0.61	0.61
73	0.61	0.62	0.62	0.62	0.63	0.63	0.63	0.63	0.64	0.64
74	0.64	0.65	0.65	0.65	0.66	0.66	0.66	0.67	0.67	0.67
75	0.67	0.68	0.68	0.68	0.69	0.69	0.69	0.70	0.70	0.70
76	0.71	0.71	0.71	0.72	0.72	0.72	0.73	0.73	0.73	0.74
77	0.74	0.74	0.75	0.75	0.75	0.76	0.76	0.76	0.77	0.77
78	0.77	0.78	0.78	0.78	0.79	0.79	0.79	0.80	0.80	0.80
79	0.81	0.81	0.81	0.82	0.82	0.82	0.83	0.83	0.83	0.84
80	0.84	0.85	0.85	0.85	0.86	0.86	0.86	0.87	0.87	0.87
81	0.88	0.88	0.89	0.89	0.89	0.90	0.90	0.90	0.91	0.91
82	0.92	0.92	0.92	0.93	0.93	0.93	0.94	0.94	0.95	0.95
83	0.95	0.96	0.96	0.97	0.97	0.97	0.98	0.98	0.99	0.99
84	0.99	1.00	1.00	1.01	1.01	1.02	1.02	1.02	1.03	1.03
85	1.04	1.04	1.05	1.05	1.05	1.06	1.06	1.07	1.07	1.08
86	1.08	1.08	1.09	1.09	1.10	1.10	1.11	1.11	1.12	1.12
87	1.13	1.13	1.14	1.14	1.15	1.15	1.16	1.16	1.17	1.17
88	1.18	1.18	1.19	1.19	1.20	1.20	1.21	1.21	1.22	1.22
89	1.23	1.23	1.24	1.24	1.25	1.25	1.26	1.26	1.27	1.28
90	1.28	1.29	1.29	1.30	1.30	1.31	1.32	1.32	1.33	1.33
91	1.34	1.35	1.35	1.36	1.37	1.37	1.38	1.39	1.39	1.40
92	1.41	1.41	1.42	1.43	1.43	1.44	1.45	1.45	1.46	1.47
93	1.48	1.48	1.49	1.50	1.51	1.51	1.52	1.53	1.54	1.55
94	1.55	1.56	1.57	1.58	1.59	1.60	1.61	1.62	1.63	1.64
95	1.64	1.65	1.66	1.67	1.68	1.70	1.71	1.72	1.73	1.74
96	1.75	1.76	1.77	1.79	1.80	1.81	1.83	1.84	1.85	1.87
97	1.88	1.90	1.91	1.93	1.94	1.96	1.98	2.00	2.01	2.03
98	2.05	2.07	2.10	2.12	2.14	2.17	2.20	2.23	2.26	2.29
99	2.33	2.37	2.41	2.46	2.51	2.58	2.65	2.75	2.88	3.09

Table A7 Critical values for the Wilcoxon matched pairs signed rank test.

Reproduced from Table 21 of White *et al.* (1979) with permission of authors and publishers.

N = number of non-zero differences
T = smaller of T_+ and T_-
Significant if $T <$ critical value

	One-sided P value			
	0.05	0.025	0.01	0.005
	Two-sided P value			
N	0.1	0.05	0.02	0.01
5	1			
6	2	1		
7	4	2	0	
8	6	4	2	0
9	8	6	3	2
10	11	8	5	3
11	14	11	7	5
12	17	14	10	7
13	21	17	13	10
14	26	21	16	13
15	30	25	20	16
16	36	30	24	19
17	41	35	28	23
18	47	40	33	28
19	54	46	38	32
20	60	52	43	37
21	68	59	49	43
22	75	66	56	49
23	83	73	62	55
24	92	81	69	61
25	101	90	77	68
26	110	98	85	76
27	120	107	93	84
28	130	117	102	92
29	141	127	111	100
30	152	137	120	109
31	163	148	130	118
32	175	159	141	128
33	188	171	151	138
34	201	183	162	149
35	214	195	174	160
36	228	208	186	171
37	242	222	198	183
38	256	235	211	195
39	271	250	224	208
40	287	264	238	221
41	303	279	252	234
42	319	295	267	248
43	336	311	281	262
44	353	327	297	277
45	371	344	313	292
46	389	361	329	307
47	408	397	345	323
48	427	397	362	339
49	446	415	380	356
50	466	434	398	373

Table A8 Critical ranges for the Wilcoxon rank sum test.

Reproduced from Table A7 of Cotton (1974) with permission of the author and publishers.

n_1, n_2 = sample sizes of two groups
T = sum of ranks in group with smaller sample size
Significant if T on boundaries or outside critical range

	One-sided P value		
	0.025	0.005	0.0005
	Two-sided P value		
n_1, n_2	0.05	0.01	0.001
2, 8	3, 19		
2, 9	3, 21		
2, 10	3, 23		
2, 11	4, 24		
2, 12	4, 26		
2, 13	4, 28		
2, 14	4, 30		
2, 15	4, 32		
2, 16	4, 34		
2, 17	5, 35		
2, 18	5, 37		
2, 19	5, 39	3, 41	
2, 20	5, 41	3, 43	
2, 21	6, 42	3, 45	
2, 22	6, 44	3, 47	
2, 23	6, 46	3, 49	
2, 24	6, 48	3, 51	
2, 25	6, 50	3, 53	
3, 5	6, 21		
3, 6	7, 23		
3, 7	7, 26		
3, 8	8, 28		
3, 9	8, 31	6, 33	
3, 10	9, 33	6, 36	
3, 11	9, 36	6, 39	
3, 12	10, 38	7, 41	
3, 13	10, 41	7, 44	
3, 14	11, 43	7, 47	
3, 15	11, 46	8, 49	
3, 16	12, 48	8, 52	
3, 17	12, 51	8, 55	
3, 18	13, 53	8, 58	
3, 19	13, 56	9, 60	
3, 20	14, 58	9, 63	
3, 21	14, 61	9, 66	6, 69
3, 22	15, 63	10, 68	6, 72
3, 23	15, 66	10, 71	6, 75
3, 24	16, 68	10, 74	6, 78
3, 25	19, 71	11, 76	6, 81
4, 4	10, 26		
4, 5	11, 29		
4, 6	12, 32	10, 34	
4, 7	13, 35	10, 38	
4, 8	14, 38	11, 41	
4, 9	15, 41	11, 45	
4, 10	15, 45	12, 48	
4, 11	16, 48	12, 52	
4, 12	17, 51	13, 55	
4, 13	18, 54	14, 58	10, 62
4, 14	19, 57	14, 62	10, 66
4, 15	20, 60	15, 65	10, 70
4, 16	21, 63	15, 69	11, 73
4, 17	21, 67	16, 72	11, 77
4, 18	22, 70	16, 76	11, 81
4, 19	23, 73	17, 79	12, 84
4, 20	24, 76	18, 82	12, 88
4, 21	25, 79	18, 86	12, 92
4, 22	26, 82	19, 89	13, 95
4, 23	27, 85	19, 93	13, 99
4, 24	28, 88	20, 96	13, 103
4, 25	28, 92	20, 100	14, 106
5, 5	17, 38	15, 40	
5, 6	18, 42	16, 44	
5, 7	20, 45	17, 48	
5, 8	21, 49	17, 53	
5, 9	22, 53	18, 57	15, 60
5, 10	23, 57	19, 61	15, 65
5, 11	24, 61	20, 65	16, 69
5, 12	26, 64	21, 69	16, 74
5, 13	27, 68	22, 73	17, 78
5, 14	28, 72	22, 78	17, 83
5, 15	29, 76	23, 82	18, 87
5, 16	31, 79	24, 86	18, 92
5, 17	32, 83	25, 90	19, 96
5, 18	33, 87	26, 94	19, 101
5, 19	34, 91	27, 98	20, 105
5, 20	35, 95	28, 102	20, 110
5, 21	37, 98	29, 106	21, 114
5, 22	38, 102	29, 111	21, 119
5, 23	39, 106	30, 115	22, 123
5, 24	40, 110	31, 119	23, 127
5, 25	42, 113	32, 123	23, 132
6, 6	26, 52	23, 55	
6, 7	27, 57	24, 60	
6, 8	29, 61	25, 65	21, 69
6, 9	31, 65	26, 70	22, 74
6, 10	32, 70	27, 75	23, 79
6, 11	34, 74	28, 80	23, 85
6, 12	35, 79	30, 84	24, 90
6, 13	37, 83	31, 89	25, 95

Table A8 *continued*

	One-sided *P* value		
	0.025	0.005	0.0005
	Two-sided *P* value		
n_1, n_2	0.05	0.01	0.001
6, 14	38, 88	32, 94	26, 100
6, 15	40, 92	33, 99	26, 106
6, 16	42, 96	34, 104	27, 111
6, 17	43, 101	36, 108	28, 116
6, 18	45, 105	37, 113	29, 121
6, 19	46, 110	38, 118	29, 127
6, 20	48, 114	39, 123	30, 132
6, 21	50, 118	40, 128	31, 137
6, 22	51, 123	42, 132	32, 142
6, 23	53, 127	43, 137	33, 147
6, 24	55, 131	44, 142	34, 152
7, 7	36, 69	32, 73	28, 77
7, 8	38, 74	34, 78	29, 83
7, 9	40, 79	35, 84	30, 89
7, 10	42, 84	37, 89	31, 95
7, 11	44, 89	38, 95	32, 101
7, 12	46, 94	40, 100	33, 107
7, 13	48, 99	41, 106	34, 113
7, 14	50, 104	43, 111	35, 119
7, 15	52, 109	44, 117	36, 125
7, 16	54, 114	46, 122	37, 131
7, 17	56, 119	47, 128	38, 137
7, 18	58, 124	49, 133	39, 143
7, 19	60, 129	50, 139	41, 148
7, 20	62, 134	52, 144	42, 154
7, 21	64, 139	53, 150	43, 160
7, 22	66, 144	55, 155	44, 166
7, 23	68, 149	57, 160	45, 172
8, 8	49, 87	43, 93	38, 98
8, 9	51, 93	45, 99	40, 104
8, 10	53, 99	47, 105	41, 111
8, 11	55, 105	49, 111	42, 118
8, 12	58, 110	51, 117	43, 125
8, 13	60, 116	53, 123	45, 131
8, 14	63, 121	54, 130	46, 138
8, 15	65, 127	56, 136	47, 145
8, 16	67, 133	58, 142	49, 151
8, 17	70, 138	60, 148	50, 158
8, 18	72, 144	62, 154	51, 165
8, 19	74, 150	64, 160	53, 171
8, 20	77, 155	66, 166	54, 178
8, 21	79, 161	68, 172	56, 184
8, 22	82, 166	70, 178	57, 191
9, 9	63, 108	56, 115	50, 121
9, 10	65, 115	58, 122	52, 128
9, 11	68, 121	61, 128	53, 136
9, 12	71, 127	63, 135	55, 143

	One-sided *P* value		
	0.025	0.005	0.0005
	Two-sided *P* value		
n_1, n_2	0.05	0.01	0.001
9, 13	73, 134	65, 142	56, 151
9, 14	76, 140	67, 149	58, 158
9, 15	79, 146	70, 155	60, 165
9, 16	82, 152	72, 162	61, 173
9, 17	84, 159	74, 169	63, 180
9, 18	87, 165	76, 176	65, 187
9, 19	90, 171	78, 183	66, 195
9, 20	93, 177	81, 189	68, 202
9, 21	95, 184	83, 196	70, 209
10, 10	78, 132	71, 139	63, 147
10, 11	81, 139	74, 146	65, 155
10, 12	85, 145	76, 154	67, 163
10, 13	88, 152	79, 161	69, 171
10, 14	91, 159	81, 169	71, 179
10, 15	94, 166	84, 176	73, 187
10, 16	97, 173	86, 184	75, 195
10, 17	100, 180	89, 191	77, 203
10, 18	103, 187	92, 198	79, 211
10, 19	107, 193	94, 206	81, 219
10, 20	110, 200	97, 213	83, 227
11, 11	96, 157	87, 166	78, 175
11, 12	99, 165	90, 174	81, 183
11, 13	103, 172	93, 182	83, 192
11, 14	106, 180	96, 190	85, 201
11, 15	110, 187	99, 198	87, 210
11, 16	114, 194	102, 206	90, 218
11, 17	117, 202	105, 214	92, 227
11, 18	121, 209	108, 222	94, 236
11, 19	124, 217	111, 230	97, 244
12, 12	115, 185	106, 194	95, 205
12, 13	119, 193	109, 203	98, 214
12, 14	123, 201	112, 212	100, 224
12, 15	127, 209	115, 221	103, 233
12, 16	131, 217	119, 229	105, 243
12, 17	135, 225	122, 238	108, 252
12, 18	139, 233	125, 247	111, 261
13, 13	137, 214	125, 226	114, 237
13, 14	141, 223	129, 235	116, 248
13, 15	145, 232	133, 244	119, 258
13, 16	150, 240	137, 253	122, 268
13, 17	154, 249	140, 263	125, 278
14, 14	160, 246	147, 259	134, 272
14, 15	164, 256	151, 269	137, 283
14, 16	169, 265	155, 279	140, 294
15, 15	185, 280	171, 294	156, 309

Table A9 Critical values of the Spearman rank correlation coefficient.

Significant if $r_s >$ critical value. Adapted from Table A8 of Colton (1974) and from Table 17 of White *et al.* (1979) with permission of the authors and publishers.

No. of pairs	Two-sided *P* value 0.05	Two-sided *P* value 0.01	One-sided *P* value 0.05	One-sided *P* value 0.01
5	—	—	0.900	—
6	0.886	—	0.829	0.943
7	0.786	—	0.714	0.893
8	0.738	0.881	0.643	0.833
9	0.683	0.833	0.600	0.783
10	0.648	0.794	0.564	0.746
12	0.591	0.780	0.506	0.712
14	0.545	0.716	0.456	0.645
16	0.507	0.666	0.425	0.601
18	0.476	0.625	0.399	0.564
20	0.450	0.591	0.377	0.534
22	0.428	0.562	0.359	0.508
24	0.409	0.537	0.343	0.485
26	0.392	0.515	0.329	0.465
28	0.377	0.496	0.317	0.448
30	0.364	0.478	0.306	0.432

Table A10 Random numbers.

Reproduced from Table XXXIII of Fisher and Yates (1963) following Armitage (1971) by permission of authors and publishers.

03 47 43 73 86	36 96 47 36 61	46 98 63 71 62	33 26 16 80 45	60 11 14 10 95
97 74 24 67 62	42 81 14 57 20	42 53 32 37 32	27 07 36 07 51	24 51 79 89 73
16 76 62 27 66	56 50 26 71 07	32 90 79 78 53	13 55 38 58 59	88 97 54 14 10
12 56 85 99 26	96 96 68 27 31	05 03 72 93 15	57 12 10 14 21	88 26 49 81 76
55 59 56 35 64	38 54 82 46 22	31 62 43 09 90	06 18 44 32 53	23 83 01 30 30
16 22 77 94 39	49 54 43 54 82	17 37 93 23 78	87 35 20 96 43	84 26 34 91 64
84 42 17 53 31	57 24 55 06 88	77 04 74 47 67	21 76 33 50 25	83 92 12 06 76
63 01 63 78 59	16 95 55 67 19	98 10 50 71 75	12 86 73 58 07	44 39 52 38 79
33 21 12 34 29	78 64 56 07 82	52 42 07 44 38	15 51 00 13 42	99 66 02 79 54
57 60 86 32 44	09 47 27 96 54	49 17 46 09 62	90 52 84 77 27	08 02 73 43 28
18 18 07 92 46	44 17 16 58 09	79 83 86 19 62	06 76 50 03 10	55 23 64 05 05
26 62 38 97 75	84 16 07 44 99	83 11 46 32 24	20 14 85 88 45	10 93 72 88 71
23 42 40 64 74	82 97 77 77 81	07 45 32 14 08	32 98 94 07 72	93 85 79 10 75
52 36 28 19 95	50 92 26 11 97	00 56 76 31 38	80 22 02 53 53	86 60 42 04 53
37 85 94 35 12	83 39 50 08 30	42 34 07 96 88	54 42 06 87 98	35 85 29 48 39
70 29 17 12 13	40 33 20 38 26	13 89 51 03 74	17 76 37 13 04	07 74 21 19 30
56 62 18 37 35	96 83 50 87 75	97 12 25 93 47	70 33 24 03 54	97 77 46 44 80
99 49 57 22 77	88 42 95 45 72	16 64 36 16 00	04 43 18 66 79	94 77 24 21 90
16 08 15 04 72	33 27 14 34 09	45 59 34 68 49	12 72 07 34 45	99 27 72 95 14
31 16 93 32 43	50 27 89 87 19	20 15 37 00 49	52 85 66 60 44	38 68 88 11 80
68 34 30 13 70	55 74 30 77 40	44 22 78 84 26	04 33 46 09 52	68 07 97 06 57
74 57 25 65 76	59 29 97 68 60	71 91 38 67 54	13 58 18 24 76	15 54 55 95 52
27 42 37 86 53	48 55 90 65 72	96 57 69 36 10	96 46 92 42 45	97 60 49 04 91
00 39 68 29 61	66 37 32 20 30	77 84 57 03 29	10 45 65 04 26	11 04 96 67 24
29 94 98 94 24	68 49 69 10 82	53 75 91 93 30	34 25 20 57 27	40 48 73 51 92

Table A10 Random numbers *continued*

16 90 82 66 59	83 62 64 11 12	67 19 00 71 74	60 47 21 29 68	02 02 37 03 31
11 27 94 75 06	06 09 19 74 66	02 94 37 34 02	76 70 90 30 86	38 45 94 30 38
35 24 10 16 20	33 32 51 26 38	79 78 45 04 91	16 92 53 56 16	02 75 50 95 98
38 23 16 86 38	42 38 97 01 50	87 75 66 81 41	40 01 74 91 62	48 51 84 08 32
31 96 25 91 47	96 44 33 49 13	34 86 82 53 91	00 52 43 48 85	27 55 26 89 62
66 67 40 67 14	64 05 71 95 86	11 05 65 09 68	76 83 20 37 90	57 16 00 11 66
14 90 84 45 11	75 73 88 05 90	52 27 41 14 86	22 98 12 22 08	07 52 74 95 80
68 05 51 18 00	33 96 02 75 19	07 60 62 93 55	59 33 82 43 90	49 37 38 44 59
20 46 78 73 90	97 51 40 14 02	04 02 33 31 08	39 54 16 49 36	47 95 93 13 30
64 19 58 97 79	15 06 15 93 20	01 90 10 75 06	40 78 78 89 62	02 67 74 17 33
05 26 93 70 60	22 35 85 15 13	92 03 51 59 77	59 56 78 06 83	52 91 05 70 74
07 97 10 88 23	09 98 42 99 64	61 71 62 99 15	06 51 29 16 93	58 05 77 09 51
68 71 86 85 85	54 87 66 47 54	73 32 08 11 12	44 95 92 63 16	29 56 24 29 48
26 99 61 65 53	58 37 78 80 70	42 10 50 67 42	32 17 55 85 74	94 44 67 16 94
14 65 52 68 75	87 59 36 22 41	26 78 63 06 55	13 08 27 01 50	15 29 39 39 43
17 53 77 58 71	71 41 61 50 72	12 41 94 96 26	44 95 27 36 99	02 96 74 30 83
90 26 59 21 19	23 52 23 33 12	96 93 02 18 39	07 02 18 36 07	25 99 32 70 23
41 23 52 55 99	31 04 49 69 96	10 47 48 45 88	13 41 43 89 20	97 17 14 49 17
60 20 50 81 69	31 99 73 68 68	35 81 33 03 76	24 30 12 48 60	18 99 10 72 34
91 25 38 05 90	94 58 28 41 36	45 37 59 03 09	90 35 57 29 12	82 62 54 65 60
34 50 57 74 37	98 80 33 00 91	09 77 93 19 82	74 94 80 04 04	45 07 31 66 49
85 22 04 39 43	73 81 53 94 79	33 62 46 86 28	08 31 54 46 31	53 94 13 38 47
09 79 13 77 48	73 82 97 22 21	05 03 27 24 83	72 89 44 05 60	35 80 39 94 88
88 75 80 18 14	22 95 75 42 49	39 32 82 22 49	02 48 07 70 37	16 04 61 67 87
90 96 23 70 00	39 00 03 06 90	55 85 78 38 36	94 37 30 69 32	90 89 00 76 33

53	74	23	99	67	61	32	28	69	84	94	62	67	86	24	98	33	41	19	95	47	53	53	38	09
63	38	06	86	54	99	00	65	26	94	02	82	90	23	07	79	62	67	80	60	75	91	12	81	19
35	30	58	21	46	06	72	17	10	94	25	21	31	75	96	49	28	24	00	49	55	65	79	78	07
63	43	36	82	69	65	51	18	37	88	61	38	44	12	45	32	92	85	88	65	54	34	81	85	35
98	25	37	55	26	01	91	82	81	46	74	71	12	94	97	24	02	71	37	07	03	92	18	66	75
02	63	21	17	69	71	50	80	89	56	38	15	70	11	48	43	40	45	86	98	00	83	26	91	03
64	55	22	21	82	48	22	28	06	00	61	54	13	43	91	82	78	12	23	29	06	66	24	12	27
85	07	26	13	89	01	10	07	82	04	59	63	69	36	03	69	11	15	83	80	13	29	54	19	28
58	54	16	24	15	51	54	44	82	00	62	61	65	04	69	38	18	65	18	97	85	72	13	49	21
34	85	27	84	87	61	48	64	56	26	90	18	48	13	26	37	70	15	42	57	65	65	80	39	07
03	92	18	27	46	57	99	16	96	56	30	33	72	85	22	84	64	38	56	98	99	01	30	98	64
62	95	30	27	59	37	75	41	66	48	86	97	80	61	45	23	53	04	01	63	45	76	08	64	27
08	45	93	15	22	60	21	75	46	91	98	77	27	85	42	28	88	61	08	84	69	62	03	42	73
07	08	55	18	40	45	44	75	13	90	24	94	96	61	02	57	55	66	83	15	73	42	37	11	61
01	85	89	95	66	51	10	19	34	88	15	84	97	19	75	12	76	39	43	78	64	63	91	08	25
72	84	71	14	35	19	11	58	49	26	50	11	17	17	76	86	31	57	20	18	95	60	78	46	75
88	78	28	16	84	13	52	53	94	53	75	45	69	30	96	73	89	65	70	31	99	17	43	48	76
45	17	75	65	57	28	40	19	72	12	25	12	74	75	67	60	40	60	81	19	24	62	01	61	16
96	76	28	12	54	22	01	11	94	25	71	96	16	16	88	68	64	36	74	45	19	59	50	88	92
43	31	67	72	30	24	02	94	08	63	38	32	36	66	02	69	36	38	25	39	48	03	45	15	22
50	44	66	44	21	66	06	58	05	62	68	15	54	35	02	42	35	48	96	32	14	52	41	52	48
22	66	22	15	86	26	63	75	41	99	58	42	36	72	24	58	37	52	18	51	03	37	18	39	11
96	24	40	14	51	23	22	30	88	57	95	67	47	29	83	94	69	40	06	07	18	16	36	78	86
31	73	91	61	19	60	20	72	93	48	98	57	07	23	69	65	95	39	69	58	56	80	30	19	44
78	60	73	99	84	43	89	94	36	45	56	69	47	07	41	90	22	91	07	12	78	35	34	08	72

Table A10 Random numbers *continued*

84	37	90	61	56	70	10	23	98	05	85	11	34	76	60	76	48	45	34	60	01	64	18	39	96
36	67	10	08	23	98	93	35	08	86	99	29	76	29	81	33	34	91	58	93	63	14	52	32	52
07	28	59	07	48	89	64	58	89	75	83	85	62	27	89	30	14	78	56	27	86	63	59	80	02
10	15	83	87	60	79	24	31	66	56	21	48	24	06	93	91	98	94	05	49	01	47	59	38	00
55	19	68	97	65	03	73	52	16	56	00	53	55	90	27	33	42	29	38	87	22	13	88	83	34
53	81	29	13	39	35	01	20	71	34	62	33	74	82	14	53	73	19	09	03	56	54	29	56	93
51	86	32	68	92	33	98	74	66	99	40	14	71	94	58	45	94	19	38	81	14	44	99	81	07
35	91	70	29	13	80	03	54	07	27	96	94	78	32	66	50	95	52	74	33	13	80	55	62	54
37	71	67	95	13	20	02	44	95	94	64	85	04	05	72	01	32	90	76	14	53	89	74	60	41
93	66	13	83	27	92	79	64	64	72	28	54	96	53	84	48	14	52	98	94	56	07	93	89	30
02	96	08	45	65	13	05	00	41	84	93	07	54	72	59	21	45	57	09	77	19	48	56	27	44
49	83	43	48	35	82	88	33	69	96	72	36	04	19	76	47	45	15	18	60	82	11	08	95	97
84	60	71	62	46	40	80	81	30	37	34	39	23	05	38	25	15	35	71	30	88	12	57	21	77
18	17	30	88	71	44	91	14	88	47	89	23	30	63	15	56	34	20	47	89	99	82	93	24	98
79	69	10	61	78	71	32	76	95	62	87	00	22	58	40	92	54	01	75	25	43	11	71	99	31
75	93	36	57	83	56	20	14	82	11	74	21	97	90	65	96	42	68	63	86	74	54	13	26	94
38	30	92	29	03	06	28	81	39	38	62	25	06	84	63	61	29	08	93	67	04	32	92	08	09
51	29	50	10	34	31	57	75	95	80	51	97	02	74	77	76	15	48	49	44	18	55	63	77	09
21	31	38	86	24	37	79	81	53	74	73	24	16	10	33	52	83	90	94	76	70	47	14	54	36
29	01	23	87	88	58	02	39	37	67	42	10	14	20	92	16	55	23	42	45	54	96	09	11	06
95	33	95	22	00	18	74	72	00	18	38	79	58	69	32	81	76	80	26	92	82	80	84	25	39
90	84	60	79	80	24	36	59	87	38	82	07	53	89	35	96	35	23	79	18	05	98	90	07	35
46	40	62	98	82	54	97	20	56	95	15	74	80	08	32	16	46	70	50	80	67	72	16	42	79
20	31	89	03	43	38	46	82	68	72	32	14	82	99	70	80	60	47	18	97	63	49	30	21	30
71	59	73	05	50	08	22	23	71	77	91	01	93	20	49	82	96	59	26	94	66	39	67	98	60

Bibliography

General

Anderson S., Auquier A., Hauck W.W., Oakes D., Vandaele W. & Weisberg H.I. (1980) *Statistical Methods for Comparative Studies.* John Wiley & Sons, New York.

Armitage P. & Berry G. (1987) *Statistical Methods in Medical Research*, 2nd edition. Blackwell Scientific Publications, Oxford.

Bradford Hill A. (1984) *A Short Textbook of Medical Statistics*, 11th edition. Hodder & Stoughton, London.

Cochran W.G. (1954) Some methods for strengthening the common χ^2 tests. *Biometrics* **10**, 417–51.

Colton T. (1974) *Statistics in Medicine.* Little, Brown & Co., Boston.

Dobson A.J. (1983) *An Introduction to Statistical Modelling.* Chapman & Hall, London.

GLIM (1978) Numerical Algorithms Group, Oxford.

Huitson A. (1980) *The Analysis of Variance: A Basic Course.* Charles Griffin & Co., London.

Kirkwood T.B.L. (1979) Geometric means and measures of dispersion. *Biometrics* **35**, 908–9.

Lindley D.V. (1965) *Introduction to Probability and Statistics from a Bayesian Viewpoint. Part 1, Probability. Part 2, Inference.* Cambridge University Press, Cambridge.

Oldham P.D. (1968) *Measurement in Medicine: the Interpretation of Numerical Data.* English Universities Press, London.

Siegel S. (1956) *Non-parametric Statisties for the Behavioural Sciences.* McGraw-Hill Kogakusha Ltd., Tokyo.

Sampling methods

Cochran W.G. (1977) *Sampling Techniques*, 3rd edition. John Wiley & Sons, New York.

Lutz W. (1986) *Survey Sampling*, 2nd edition. International Epidemiological Association, Geneva.

Moser C. & Kalton G. (1971) *Survey Methods in Social Investigation*, 2nd edition. Heinemann Educational Books, London.

Stuart A. (1984) *The Ideas of Sampling* (Griffin's Statistical Monographs and Course Series, No. 4). Charles Griffin & Co., High Wycombe.

Survival analysis

Cox D.R. & Oakes D. (1984) *Analysis of Survival Data.* Chapman & Hall, London.

Peto R., Pike M.C., Armitage P., Breslow N.E., Cox D.R., Howard S.V., Mantel N., McPherson K., Peto J. & Smith P.G. (1976) Design and analysis of randomized clinical trials requiring prolonged observation of each patient. I. Introduction and design. *British Journal of Cancer* **34**, 585–612.

Peto R., Pike M.C., Armitage P., Breslow N.E., Cox D.R., Howard S.V., Mantel N., McPherson K., Peto J. & Smith P.G. (1977) Design and analysis of randomized clinical trials requiring prolonged observation of each patient. II. Analysis and examples. *British Journal of Cancer* **35**, 1–39.

Clinical trials

Armitage P. (1975) *Sequential Medical Trials*, 2nd edition. Blackwell Scientific Publications, Oxford.

Cancer Research Campaign Working Party in Breast Conservation (1983) Informed consent: ethical, legal, and medical implications for doctors and patients who participate in randomised clinical trials. *British Medical Journal* **286,** 1117–21.

Pocock S.J. (1983) *Clinical Trials: a Practical Approach.* John Wiley & Sons, Chichester.

Epidemiology

Breslow N.E. & Day N.E. (1980) *Statistical Methods in Cancer Research Volume 1—The Analysis of Case–Control Studies.* International Agency for Research on Cancer, Lyon.

Kleinbaum D.G., Kupper L.L. & Morgenstern H. (1982) *Epidemiologic Research: Principles and Quantitative Methods.* Van Nostrand Reinhold, New York.

Lilienfeld A.M. & Lilienfeld D.E. (1980) *Foundations of Epidemiology*, 2nd edition. Oxford University Press, New York.

Rothman K.J. (1986) *Modern Epidemiology.* Little, Brown & Co., Boston.

Schlesselman J.J. (1982) *Case–Control Studies: Design, Conduct, Analysis.* Oxford University Press, New York.

Smith P.G. (1982) Spatial and temporal clustering. In *Cancer Epidemiology and Prevention* (eds Schottenfeld D. & Fraumeni J.F.). W.B. Saunders, Philadelphia.

Smith P.G. (1987) Evaluating interventions against tropical diseases. *International Journal of Epidemiology* **16,** 159–66.

Smith P.G., Rodrigues L.C. & Fine P.E.M. (1984) Assessment of the protective efficacy of vaccines against common diseases using case–control and cohort studies. *International Journal of Epidemiology* **13,** 87–93.

Vandenbrouke J.P. (1985) On the rediscovery of a distinction. *American Journal of Epidemiology* **121,** 627–8.

Statistical tables

Fisher R.A. & Yates F. (1963) *Statistical Tables for Biological, Agricultural and Medical Research*, 6th Edition. Oliver & Boyd, Edinburgh.

Geigy Scientific Tables, Volume 2 (1982). Ciba-Geigy, Basle.

Pearson E.S. & Hartley H.O. (1966) *Biometrika Tables for Statisticians*, Volume 1, 3rd Edition. Cambridge University Press.

White J., Yeats A. & Skipworth G. (1979) *Tables for Statisticians*, 3rd Edition. Stanley Thornes, Cheltenham.

Index